http://www

Praise for
Leanne Shirtliffe and *Don't Lick the Minivan*

"Leanne Shirtliffe is awesome and so is this book. I'm bad at writing blurbs."

> —Jenny Lawson (The Bloggess), *New York Times* bestselling author of *Let's Pretend This Never Happened*

"Toddler diarrhea and newborn vomit aren't all that entertaining, but somehow when Leanne Shirtliffe writes about it, it's laugh-out-loud funny. I swear, she's living in my house and taking notes. Actually, I wish she were—we'd have a freaking blast together."

> —Jill Smokler, *New York Times* bestselling author of *Confessions of a Scary Mommy*

"When you become a parent, conversations start to sound more like a game of Mad Libs than anything actually sane. In the laugh-out-loud book *Don't Lick the Minivan*, Leanne Shirtliffe shares the funniest phrases she never thought she'd say. Hands down, the best book with the phrase 'He looks like a human Pez dispenser' I've read all year!"

> —Kristen Pomranz, Editor, Nickelodeon's NickMom.com

"Leanne Shirtliffe has a sharp eye for the little moments of insanity that make up the modern parenting experience. Also, she's super funny and the chapters are short enough to read in the four minutes you're allowed in the bathroom each day."

> —Stefanie Wilder-Taylor, bestselling author of *Sippy Cups Are Not for Chardonnay* and *Naptime Is the New Happy Hour*

"Forget about the darndest things that kids say, it's what comes out of our own mouths when we become parents that's the real shocker. Leanne has a way of making us see the humor in the exchanges we have with our kids, our friends, and most importantly, ourselves. Her quick and witty writing style is the perfect antidote for all moms suffering through life's most unfunny moments with our kids."

—Kathy Buckworth, author of *Shut Up and Eat* and *The BlackBerry Diaries*

"Leanne Shirtliffe has written a side-splitting and thoughtful take on life with twins. As a humor writer, a parent, and a twin myself, this book had me laughing and thinking, then laughing again, long after I finished it. If you're into public fits of hysterics, try reading this book on a subway or bus, and prepare for strange looks from fellow passengers."

—Terry Fallis, author of *The Best Laid Plans* and winner of both The Stephen Leacock Award for Humour and Canada Reads 2011

"Leanne Shirtliffe provides a heartfelt, honest, and hilarious journey through parenthood in this high-flying family love letter, cautionary how-to, and what's-got-to-be-a-pro-vasectomy screed. After achieving Zen through laughter, you'll wish you were her, be glad you're not, and order two more shots."

—Jeff Kreisler, writer for Comedy Central and author of the bestselling *Get Rich Cheating*

"From forgetting your kid's . . . um . . . name, to packing an 'eco-friendly lunch' (by de-plasticizing the individually wrapped cheese sticks at home), this book had me realizing: All us parents are partners in absurdity. And that's a good thing!"

—Lenore Skenazy, author of *Free-Range Kids: How to Raise Safe Self-Reliant Children (Without Going Nuts with Worry)*

DON'T
LICK THE
MINIVAN

DON'T LICK THE MINIVAN

AND OTHER THINGS I NEVER THOUGHT I'D SAY TO MY KIDS

LEANNE SHIRTLIFFE

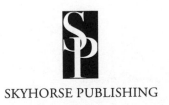

SKYHORSE PUBLISHING

Skyhorse Publishing books may be purchased in bulk at special discounts for sales promotion, corporate gifts, fund-raising, educational purposes, or Colin Firth groupies. Special editions can also be created to specifications. For details, contact the Special Sales Department, Skyhorse Publishing, 307 West 36th Street, 11th Floor, New York, NY 10018 or info@skyhorsepublishing.com.

Skyhorse® and Skyhorse Publishing® are registered trademarks of Skyhorse Publishing, Inc.®, a Delaware corporation.

Visit our website at www.skyhorsepublishing.com.

10 9 8 7 6 5 4 3 2 1

Library of Congress Cataloging-in-Publication Data
Shirtliffe, Leanne.
 Don't lick the minivan, and other things I never thought I'd say to my kids /
Leanne Shirtliffe.
    pages cm
 ISBN 978-1-62087-526-1 (hardcover : alk. paper) 1. Parenting--Humor. I.
Title.
 PN6231.P2S55 2013
 818'.607--dc23

                                2012047599

Printed in the United States of America

For C and VW,
You three make me laugh like no one else.
Thank you.

For my children's future therapist(s),
You're welcome.

"Having a baby is like suddenly
getting the world's worst roommate,
like having Janis Joplin
with a bad hangover and PMS
come to stay with you."

~Anne Lamott

"There are two things in life
for which we are
never truly prepared:
twins."

~Josh Billings

CONTENTS

INTRODUCTION

A Rambling Preamble, or How This Came to Be

A WORD TO THE READER, OR MORE PRECISELY, 452 WORDS TO THE READER

Don't Lick the Minivan is a work of nonfiction that my brain believed to be true when I wrote it. Keep in mind that this same brain once believed that alligators lived in toilet bowls on the Canadian Prairies.

If characters in *Don't Lick the Minivan* bear any similarities to my husband or twins, it's not a coincidence. Some names have been changed, mostly in the Acknowledgments.

A small portion (think the size of a Polly Pocket purse before you're about to vacuum it up) of the content of this book appeared on my blog back when my mom and that guy in California were the only ones who read it regularly. An even smaller portion appeared on a friend's blog.

Many nonfiction books start with a section entitled "How to Use This Book"; so does this one. Here are Ten (+1) Ways How to Use *Don't Lick the Minivan*:

1. Read it, especially after your kids have licked or carved their names into your minivan.
2. Use it as a paperweight for either your child's art projects or your unpaid bills.

3. If you hate saccharine reflections on how changed women are because of motherhood, skip "The Sappy Files" at the end of each chapter.

4. If you like saccharine reflections on how changed women are because of motherhood, read only "The Sappy Files" (don't worry—you'll be done in five minutes so you can get back to scrapbooking your child's first and second bowel movements).

5. Throw this book at your husband if he tells you that you have the stats of an NFL football player. (Note: If you bought the e-reader version, disregard.)

6. If you have anxiety, insomnia, or depression, put the book down. Call a friend and your doctor. Once you assemble your team, feel free to read this book. Or not. I understand.

7. If you're thinking of having kids, skim the book. You might as well have a sense of what's in store for you, including how hard it is to pee after a C-section.

8. If you're debating scheduling a vasectomy, you might as well be sure. Skim the book, and then make the call.

9. Place *Don't Lick the Minivan* on your bookshelf so that the cover is facing out. You'll need to fill the space after you throw out your how-to-parent-like-an-expert books.

10. If you're doing a master's degree in psychology, peruse *Don't Lick the Minivan*. You're going to need to know how to counsel my kids.

11. Finally, if you've ever told your daughter to stop licking the minivan or your son (or husband) to get the train off his penis, this book is for you.

GET THAT TRAIN OFF YOUR PENIS

There are some people who think kids say the cutest things. I'm not one of them. I mostly block out what my twins say because it's the only way to get some silence. But occasionally I do tune in, and what I hear shocks me. It's not so much what my kids say—it's what comes spewing out of my own mouth.

Like the time I said, "Get that train off your penis."

It was a typical enough I-need-a-nanny-or-booze hour. I whizzed around the kitchen packing lunches for Earth Week, which, as the preschool memo dictated, meant litter-less. Nothing like taking a horrible task and making it harder. I started unwrapping granola bars.

"Get ready for your bath," I yelled. In our house, this once was an invitation to get naked and run around with arms waving.

Before I could place two freed-from-plastic cheese sticks into containers, my twins had stripped and begun dancing in the living room, two bare butt kids doing a leprechaun jig while singing, "We're naked, we're naked, we're naked." When Vivian and William clasped hands in a Ring-Around-the-Rosie move, visions of pagan rituals à la Stonehenge flashed through my mind.

"Get upstairs," I hollered, trying to shove eight Tupperware containers into a single lunch box. One druid listened.

After I crammed the lunches into our fridge, I looked into the now silent living room and saw a bare leg near the toy table. I walked over and found William gripping his Thomas the Tank Engine firmly in hand.

"Get that train off your penis."

I blinked away images of Sir Topham Hatt leering around the corner.

And that was the moment. The moment when I realized there may be a lot of crap that comes out of your kids' butts, but when you're a parent, almost as much comes out of your mouth.

Better get the shovel.

DON'T LICK THE MINIVAN

PART ONE

PREGNANCY AND BIRTH, OR IS THIS REALLY HAPPENING?

SO THE ACCOUNTANT GOT HER AUNT TO DO SOME WOO-WOO ON OUR UNBORN BABIES?

When I got knocked up, my husband Chris and I had been living in Thailand for three years, teaching at an international school. It took what seemed to be the majority of our first year in Southeast Asia for me to find someone who could cut my hair so that it didn't look like I'd been welding while standing in a bathtub full of water. Bangkok's humidity meant that pieces of my hair flipped in every compass direction, like they were trying to escape my head.

I found a woman with curlier and nicer hair than mine.

"Who does your hair?" I asked.

"Franck."

Soon, I hunted down Franck, a French expat living in Bangkok whose name rhymed with "honk." Franck knew how to cut hair, even if his methods were unorthodox. For part of the appointment, he'd sit on his stool-with-wheels and encircle you, not unlike a kid who's discovered his parents' twirly office chair. For the end of the haircut, he'd rise and ask you to stand up, finishing off his magic while standing.

He had a good thing going. He charged Parisian prices in a developing country; desperate and frizzled expatriates emptied money from their wallets. After I became his client, a dozen of my colleagues followed.

I'd been seeing Franck for three years when my love for him temporarily faded.

"*Allo*, Leanne," he said, holding the last syllable of my name as French men do. He was always good-natured. Then I watched as his eyes squinted at me, bringing me into focus against the blinding Thai sun.

He walked over. "Your hairrr," he said. "Your hairrr look like sheet."

"What?" I said, even though I'd heard perfectly well. "My hair does not look like sheet, does it?"

"Ah. But it does. It look like sheet. Who cut deess?"

"You did."

"*Non*. Not I. I did not cut deess." He inspected the ends.

"You did. Two months ago."

"Some-ting happened den. Tell Franck de trute." He led me to his chair, which might have been electrified given what just transpired.

"Seet," he said. "And tell me."

I sat. "Well, I'm pregnant."

"Aha. So dat eez it. Dat explains it."

"It does?"

"*Bien sur*. Your hair look like sheet because you're pregnant. De body changes. De hair changes."

"But I thought your hair was supposed to look better when you're pregnant."

"Ahh, Leanne. Most women, yes. But you? *Non*."

Parenting Tip: Avoid looking in the mirror during pregnancy. Denial is an excellent strategy that will help you once your child is born.

"Can you make me look less like sheet?"

"I try," he said. He must have noticed my pout. "But pregnancy is good, Leanne, *non*?"

"It's good, Franck. It's good."

He motioned for his assistant to wash my hair.

"But please don't tell anyone," I said. "Other than my husband, you're the only one who knows."

"Leanne, I won't tell anyone your hair look like sheet."

"No, Franck," I said. "Don't tell anyone I'm pregnant. No one knows."

Franck smiled. "*Pas de problem.*"

There are things that turn my stomach more than a French man telling me I look like sheet and more than pregnancy. But being knocked up is still high on my list. It's not so much the pregnancy; it's my memory of being pregnant with twins in Thailand.

While Bangkok might be called the City of Angels, it sometimes felt more like the City of Smells. The spectrum of stenches presented a multitude of problems for pregnant me, not the least of which was eating fried rice without upchucking refried rice. I stumbled along the sidewalks, climbing two-foot curbs and dodging vendors who were hawking a variety of smelly goods ranging from deep-fried bugs to papaya with chilies. If those didn't turn my stomach, the hawkers promising pirated Celine Dion CDs or sex would.

Most days I ate at a street stall. Having lived in Bangkok for years, I knew which portable eateries were safe. Usually I'd inhale chicken fried rice or pad thai. Sometimes, however, eating held the same level of enjoyment as getting a pap smear with a frost-laden metallic torture device.

Chris often joined me for lunch, anxious to escape the world of books he lived in as the school's librarian. He'd watch me play with the remainders of my food and shift in my plastic chair. I looked over to the propane-powered barbecue on which the vendor was cooking mystery-meat-on-a-stick. I said to Chris, "If I smell any more charred flesh, I'm going to puke up my pad thai."

He picked up his empty bamboo skewer and mimed stabbing himself in the chest. I laughed.

"Feel better?" he asked.

"I feel like I'm going to puke with a smile on my face."

That day I didn't, but on other days stray dogs lapped up my second-hand offerings, adding me to the food chain.

Things didn't become much more routine when Chris and I went to my ob-gyn guy, also known as a doctor. Given that my first trimester had included some bleeding and bed rest, I panicked at any abnormality. Whenever our doctor did an ultrasound, I just wanted him to say the word "normal." Or, as he said in his accented English, "*nor-maall*" (rhymes with "sore gal").

Every few weeks, we would come armed with a paranoid couple's list of concerns and he would answer, "*Nor-maall*, completely *nor-maall*."

At one appointment, I pulled out my scroll of questions. I looked at the doctor and asked, "Is it normal to have mushrooms growing out of my armpit?"

His forehead creased. "Mushrooms?"

I raised my arm. I'd worn a sleeveless blouse, anticipating this moment. Chris shifted, unfazed at my colony of fungi. The doctor wandered over and laughed. "Those aren't mushrooms," he said. "They're polyps."

"They're what?"

"Polyps. Or skin tags. They come, they go. *Nor-maall*."

"So, they're not mushrooms?"

"No."

"Then I shouldn't stir fry them?"

"Pardon?"

"Never mind."

When we arrived home, Chris imitated me, "Doctor, I've grown a third eye and there are radishes sprouting from my ears."

"No worries," Chris continued his impression, "it's *nor-maall*."

There are a lot of things that were *nor-maall* in Thailand that wouldn't have been in North America. The Thais have some great superstitions. One is that it's bad luck to get your hair cut on Wednesday. Another is that twins are incredibly lucky. Boy/girl twins are even luckier. And if the boy is born first—as William was in our case—you're going to start crapping gold bricks. Even if we didn't go all Midas-like, several Thai maintenance staff members asked Chris to buy lottery tickets for them. They gave him money; his job was to select the tickets. Chris would have had an easier job crapping gold bricks than picking a winning lottery ticket from the blind man with the rebar cane who approached the outskirts of the school campus daily.

At some point during my pregnancy, Chris received an email from a Thai woman in the accounting department at work. He showed it to me when he arrived home.

It read:

"I HAVE ASKED MY AUNT TO LOOK FOR THE GOOD DAY FOR YOUR CHILDREN TO BE BORN. I GAVE HER YOUR AND YOUR WIFE BIRTHDAY AND SHE COMES UP WITH THE FOLLOWING DAY AND TIME:

° MAY 22 OR 24. TIME: 6:00 AM TO 1:00 PM
° JUNE 5. TIME: 6:00 AM TO 9:00 PM
° JUNE 6. TIME: 9:00 AM TO 9:00 PM
° JUNE 12. TIME: 9:00 AM TO 3:00 PM.

BEST WISHES."

I reread the email. I used my fingers to count how many weeks I'd be pregnant by those dates. I also used my toes and every other countable thing nearby.

I paused to process this epistle.

"Let me get this straight. So the accountant got her aunt to do some woo-woo on our unborn babies?"

"Yes."

"And we're supposed to give this to our doctor?"

Chris nodded. "She said it also has something to do with the moons."

"OK. But we're not giving this to our doctor, are we?"

"He's Thai. He'd likely say it's *nor-maall.*"

"We're still not giving him the list," I said.

"You win."

"Good. You know, if our babies are born on those dates, it'll be freaky." I shifted in my chair. "But if they're not, we can blame the moon for everything they do wrong for the rest of their lives."

Which is precisely what we've done.

WE'RE IN TROUBLE IF OUR DOCTOR DOESN'T KNOW HOW WOMEN DO IT

Some babes are born in the back of a taxi; some babes are conceived in the back of a taxi. Our daughter was named in the back of a taxi.

We had just taken the Skytrain, Bangkok's version of Jetson-transit, to an English-language bookstore and picked up a baby name book. Chris suggested we take a taxi home, which meant we were stuck in one of Bangkok's infamous 24-7 traffic jams.

Having been married for four years, we'd had every conversation we ever needed to have twenty-six times. So I made up a game. I'm annoying like that.

Taking the baby name book out of the bag, I said, "Pick a number between one and three hundred ninety-two."

"Seventy," Chris said.

I flipped to page seventy. "Now we each have to find a baby name we like." We scanned the names and critiqued each other's choices.

Three turns later, I said, "Three hundred seventy-seven."

I thumbed through the pages. We both said, "Vivian."

"I think we just found a girl's name," I said.

The next day, the name discussion continued. Miraculously, we were no longer in the taxi, but at home.

"How about the name 'Humphrey'?" Chris asked.

I looked at him in shock and said, "You're kidding, right?"

He said, "No, I like Humphrey."

"No way."

"But I like it. I really do."

"I don't care if it was your grandfather's name and he died in the war saving the lives of three children who went on to win the Nobel Prize for something. It's horrible."

"Come on."

"Look," I said, "I'm carrying the babies, so I have veto power. If you name our son Humphrey, I'll kill you."

Parenting Tip: Mothers have the right to exercise veto power on the selection of baby names. The Pregnancy Convention deems this to be true.

Chris shrugged. I grabbed the baby name book and opened to Humphrey.

"It means *peaceful warrior*," I said.

"See? That's nice."

"What the hell's a peaceful warrior? It's a bloody oxymoron. I think the second meaning is beat-me-up-at-school."

"You know, any name can be made fun of."

"No, it can't," I said. "Some names are above that."

"Try me," Chris said.

"What?"

"Give me a name. Any name. I'll make fun of it."

"OK, how about Zack?"

With a delay of 0.03 seconds, Chris sang, "Zack, Zack, rhymes with butt crack."

I tried another one. "Michael."

"Mike, Mike, you're a dyke."

"You've made your point," I conceded. "But I still hate Humphrey." I looked back at the book. "After the meaning, it says 'see also Onofrio and Onufrey.'"

"See what?" Chris asked.

"Onofrio and Onufrey," I said. "They're names that are similar to Humphrey. So there we go," I said, dropping comfortably into sarcasm, "if our babies are boys, we can name them Onofrio and Onufrey. Or Ono and Onu for short."

I smirked.

This time, Chris conceded. "OK, you've made your point."

Thankfully, we didn't need to register our babies' names to attend prenatal classes at Bangkok's most prestigious hospital. It was the first of three classes that some childless administrator had scheduled over the supper hour, the time of day your blood sugar crashes. When your circulatory system has nearly twice the normal blood volume, that sugar crash can be akin to free falling off a cliff. Chris and I walked into the hospital, foolishly bypassing Starbucks, and took the elevator to the ninth floor. We took a glass of sugary orange drink. Nutritional content was overrated.

After checking in, we sat on the floor in a conference room that was devoid of chairs. With seven couples against one wall and seven against the other, I wondered if we'd play a game of Red Rover as an icebreaker. A lone projector sat in the middle of the floor, like a cactus popping out of a desert. A young Thai woman—who was so small that she'd make

Angelina Jolie look like she ate McFood daily—smiled, bowed, and started the PowerPoint. I squinted, trying to differentiate the white font from its pale yellow background, and I ended up wondering if my bad vision meant I had sudden-onset gestational diabetes.

When PowerPoint #1 was finished, a woman from public relations took us on a guided tour of the ward. The first things we saw were the high-end maternity suites, complete with a bedroom, a living room, and a full-size fridge.

"Where are the *nor-maall* rooms?" I asked.

"In the other hallway," she said. "We won't be seeing them."

Next she took us to a delivery room, showcasing the overhead light dimmer.

"Turning down the lights," she explained, "takes away the pain."

Who knew it was that easy? "Remind me to give birth in the dark," I whispered to Chris.

We returned to the chair-less conference room. After introducing the physiotherapist, the tour guide informed us that we were about to experience her favorite part. This highlight consisted of three minutes of yoga lessons, including the following instructions: "Breathe in, breathe out, shut your eyes."

Chris leaned over. "If you shut your eyes," he whispered, "it'll be dark, which means no pain."

The physiotherapist reminded us that we needed to do fifty Kegel exercises a day, which was forty more than I'd done in my life.

Two weeks later, we were back for the second prenatal class—or as the hospital called it, antenatal class. Not having spoken Latin in my past couple lifetimes, I became confused and thought this meant they were anti-birth.

No matter. I was all ears as I sat my expansive butt on the ground because the focus of this class was birthing, which sounded somewhat relevant. I was now five months along and had gained thirty-one pounds, which made sitting on the floor as comfortable as sticking a fondue fork between two vertebrae and twisting.

We began with a video entitled *Birth Is Women's Work*, a film that advocated home births. It was surreal to be sitting in a hospital hearing about natural birth, when the C-section rate at Thai private hospitals was 70 percent and rising, given my impending multiple birth C-section.

After the film, a knowledgeable, western-trained doctor explained the statistic to us, somewhat critically. Wealthy Thai women, he said, tend to request C-sections. It was a sign of prosperity, and it allowed them to select an propitious date, such as the king or queen's birthday. "That's the woo-woo part," I whispered to Chris. But it was the doctor's third reason that made me record his words verbatim. "Many women," he said, "are scared their vagina will be stretched to the extent their husbands will leave them." I was starting to see why the hospital emphasized doing Kegels and giving birth in the dark. The doctor added, "Most of the time their husbands leave them anyway." I glared at Chris. *Don't even think about it, buddy.*

The ob-gyn went on to explain that doctors also get more money for performing C-sections. Even in a prestigious private hospital, he said, doctors were only paid $240 for a normal delivery.

"Do you think we need to tip our obstetrician?" I asked Chris.

The doctor ended his message with a gentle plea to all who weren't carrying multiples—he smiled at us, knowing full well that we were stuck with a C-section—to consider natural delivery.

He ended his plea by saying, "I don't know how women do it."

I looked at Chris. "We're in trouble if our doctor doesn't know how women do it."

The doctor left, and a nurse started another PowerPoint presentation on what to expect before and during the birth or, in our case, births.

Her second slide made me pause:

ROUTINE PREPARATION
ENEMAS
SHAVING
WHAT IS IT FOR?
FOOD AND DRINKS

Chris and I started laughing.

"So," he said, "are the *Food and Drinks* related to the *shaving* or to the *enemas*?"

"No idea. Which one is preferable?" I added.

"And *what is it for*?"

We were the naughty kids with numb butts who were not much closer to figuring out how women did it.

 Parenting Tip: Misbehave during prenatal classes. Nothing is going to go according to plan anyway.

YOU THOUGHT TELLING ME I HAVE GOOD STATS FOR A FOOTBALL PLAYER WOULD BE FUNNY?

In my fifth month of pregnancy, my waist—if you could call it that—measured a whopping forty-three inches, more than a foot bigger than it did in my pre-pregnancy days. This might not seem huge, but situate me in Thailand, home to women whose waists measure in the teens, and I was Mommy Behemoth.

A friend from Texas visited around this time: a gym teacher who had a waist. As I inhaled my second order of chicken fried rice, I said, "I'm a walking Astrodome."

"You are not," she said.

"Is there a bigger stadium in Texas then?"

"Yeah, there are a few."

"Don't tell me about them."

I added sugar to my tea.

"Do you use hula hoops in your PE classes?" I continued. She paused. "Not very often."

"I don't think I could fit in a hula hoop. And I still have months to go."

I ended my masochistic rant with a sigh.

"You know," she said, "there are a lot of people who think the Astrodome is pretty nice."

I smiled.

"Well, it beats the alternative," I said. "You know, *not* getting bigger."

We spent a few lovely days together, and then she and her waist left. We wouldn't see her again until our twins were old enough to toddle off the side of a mountain.

I pored through the emails I'd fallen behind on. There was one from my cousin. My cousin and I had the luxury of being pregnant at the same time. Guilt free, we shared obscure details that would make women-with-waists—and lives—puke.

In her latest email, my cousin told me about the walk-into-the-wall contest. In our extended family, this was becoming a rite of passage. We females have been cursed/blessed with breasts like the ones boys gawked at in *National Geographic* in pre-Internet days. Consequently, when pregnant, it was a substantial milestone when your belly beat your boobs in the walk-into-the-wall contest.

I was taking the elevator to our ninth floor apartment when I thought I'd try our family litmus test. I backed up, took two Mother-May-I steps forward, and my stomach thumped the wall first. My boobs earned the second place ribbon, my nose third. My butt was dead last; I picked it up off the floor and stepped out of the elevator, which had magically stopped level with our floor. An auspicious day, indeed.

I unlocked our apartment, dropped my bag, and flopped onto the couch.

"How was your day?" Chris hollered from the kitchen.

"Great," I yelled back. "My belly is now beating my boobs in the walk-into-the-wall contest."

"The what?"

As he emerged from the kitchen with glasses of water, I explained our family contest.

"Did you do this in front of your twelfth graders?"

"No, they'd think I'm even crazier. Plus, I'd get chalk on my bump," I said. "But I'll reenact the race if you want me to."

He hadn't even answered when I took five big strides into the wall.

"Yup," he said. "The belly won."

Parenting Tip: Measure the progress of your pregnancy with the walk-into-the-wall contest. ("Progress" being a very loose term.)

I had trouble remembering pregnancy and birthing terms. Because I was teaching at the same time that I was incubating twins, I told people I was in my third *semester*, not trimester. I thought *meconium*, that black tar newborns poop out, was an element on the Periodic Table wedged somewhere between zinc and arsenic. There's a reason I'm not a chemist.

Apparently *fontanelle* was not the next trendy hotel in Vegas, but the soft spot in your newborn's cranium.

Fundal height was another term I could never remember. I originally thought it was fundus height, which soon morphed into fungus height, not surprising given the mushroom colony I had growing in my armpits.

Technically, fundal height is the measurement from the top of a woman's uterus to the tip of her pubic bone; if you're knocked up with twins, it's the length of Hollywood Boulevard.

In my thirty-sixth week of incubating, I was sitting in our Bangkok-hot apartment under a ceiling fan wearing something more than nothing, but less than clothing. More precisely, I wore a crisp cotton robe that no longer met over my belly. Our apartment was in one of Bangkok's central districts and was surrounded by other residential high rises. I estimated that 10,000 people saw me scantily clad when

I was pregnant. It was as if Ugly Naked Guy from *Friends* had migrated to Thailand for a sex change operation (a not uncommon reason for medical tourism) and was parading around my apartment. While sweating, I said to Chris, "I'm freaking huge."

"You're pregnant," he answered.

"My fungus height measures down to my ankles. Well, it would if I had ankles. Or if I could see them."

"What's your fungus height? Are those mushrooms back again?"

I looked under my arm.

"Those are long gone. I harvested them and put them in the pasta, remember?"

"So . . . fungus height?"

"Right. It's the size of my uterus."

"Lee," he said. "You're pregnant. It's normal."

Sure. *Nor-maall.*

It was Week Thirty-Seven. I wrote it down.

I had just returned from another appointment with my obstetrician where I'd been weighed by two Thai nurses whose combined mass equaled one of my thighs.

I told Chris about my weight gain and made the mistake of sharing that I now tipped the scale—quite literally—at two bills.

"Really?" he said. "Wow, with your height and weight, you have great stats for a defensive back."

I choked on my Häagen-Dazs.

"Tell me you didn't just say that out loud."

"What did I say?"

"You can't play that card. I know you remember what you said."

"It was a compliment."

I gave him the finger with the hand not holding my half-eaten ice cream. Because that's what self-help books for couples advise.

"Look," Chris continued, making the grave mistake of trying to explain himself. "DBs in the NFL are fast. They have to cover wide receivers and—"

"Wide?"

"I need to shut up, don't I?"

I pointed the now empty ice cream stick at him. "You thought telling me I have good stats for a football player would be funny?"

"Not any football player . . . a DB . . . and I thought . . . no . . . I didn't think."

 Parenting Tip: During pregnancy (or any other time), if your husband comments that you have the measurements of an NFL player, it's perfectly legal to throw this book at him.

DO YOU THINK IT'S HERETICAL IF I REFER TO MYSELF AS THE TRINITY?

In one of my pregnancy books, I read that heredity is a major determinant of whether a woman gets stretch marks during her pregnancy. I can assert with confidence that this theory has the same scientific validity as Pamela Anderson's breasts being natural.

I took more precautions to avoid getting stretch marks than I did to avoid getting pregnant. I collected lotions, potions, and emotions on my bedside table. I would've tried eye of newt and toe of frog if I didn't have to go down to Chattuchuk—Bangkok's crazy market that sells everything, including chicks dyed in primary colors (and no, I'm not talking about women, though in Bangkok, that was possible too)—to haggle for them.

Alas, all my belly rubbing was for naught. By the time I was well into my third semester, I had gained fifty pounds, and my skin stretched and turned bright purple. Easter purple. My stretch marks were well organized, seemingly etched by a city planner. They traveled in two distinct directions, avenues and streets intersecting each other on my own speed bump the size of Manhattan. My belly button was a statue lacking liberty.

Chris had the foresight not to comment on my marks. And being the good guy he is, they didn't bother him.

Whenever I bemoaned the existence of my tattooed belly, he'd shrug and go back into his mode of denial, which involved watching TV and reading.

Somewhere in the middle of a Raptors game—it was, after all, Chris Bosh's rookie season in the NBA—I sat on a chair in underwear.

"Do you want to play checkers?" I asked.

"What?" Chris answered, still looking at the TV.

"Checkers," I said. "You know, the game?"

"I know what it is," he said, eyes still focused on the Pistons's domination of the game.

"Well, do you want to play?"

"No thanks, Lee. I'm just trying to lose myself in the game."

"Are you sure?" I said. "Because I thought we could play checkers on my stretch marks."

Finally, he looked at me.

Then Vince Carter, the Raptors's star player, received a technical foul.

"#$%*!"

"I guess that's a 'no,'" I said and began looking around for tongue of dog, my latest potion.

The next night I told Chris, "You know, pregnancy should be measured in seconds."

He looked up from the serial killer novel he was reading. Evidently, the NBA had the night off.

"It should be," I continued. "I mean, they used to measure it in months. Now it's measured in weeks. If we're going for realism, it should be measured in seconds."

"You've been thinking about this."

"I've had a lot of spare seconds since I stopped working."

"You have a point," he said, trying to dismiss me so he could get back to his fictional world of carnage and ex-army badasses. I suspected this was more manageable than real life.

"In case you're wondering, nine months equals twenty-four million, one-hundred-and-ninety-two thousand seconds."

He looked up from his book. "You memorized it?"

Parenting Tip: Measure pregnancy in seconds, not weeks. It almost makes gestation seem as endless as it feels.

"Yup. I used one hundred and twenty seconds to do the math."

"Right."

"But since we're having twins, I'll likely be pregnant for a shorter time, maybe just under twenty-three million seconds."

"You didn't memorize that one?"

"Nope. Didn't want to waste any more seconds."

"Can I read my book now?"

"Sure. Go wild," I said, eyeing his book. "Jack Reacher will save the day, you know. With a toothbrush in his pocket."

"I know."

"OK."

At various times in the nine longest months of my life—usually while Chris was on his escape–reality mission—I played with words. I debated if the plural of fetus was fetuses or feti. And if it was feti, what is the plural of fetish? Could a person who was overly enamored with twins in a pregnant woman's uterus have a feti feti?

Chris, like a good husband, pretended to be amused. Together, we referred to our fetuses as Baby A and Baby B, Lefty and Righty, and Thing 1 and Thing 2.

We chose not to find out their sexes, so we had to be vague. Still, as the pregnancy dragged on we became more inventive, giving them names such as Alpha and Omega, and Engine and Caboose.

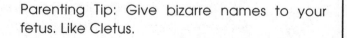

Parenting Tip: Give bizarre names to your fetus. Like Cletus.

One day, I met Chris at work and rode home with him in a *tuk tuk,* a three-wheeled motorized rickshaw that's half motorcycle, half tin can. Amid the noise and the crowded streets, I shouted, "Do you think it's heretical if I refer to myself as the Trinity?"

"The what?" Chris asked, yelling above the din of traffic and two-stroke engines.

"The Trinity," I said. "You know, the three-in-one."

He laughed. "Call yourself whatever you want," he said, rubbing my bouncing belly. "This *tuk tuk* is likely going straight to hell."

WHY DO SO MANY PEOPLE SAY STUPID THINGS TO PREGNANT WOMEN?

Before I had kids, I approached childrearing like a new project: I researched it with the goal of becoming an expert. In retrospect, this approach was as successful as a nineteen-year-old who has completed Biology 101 performing a DIY appendectomy.

I read all the books on pregnancy.

And like a good wife, I shared what I read with Chris, not caring that he was trying to multitask by watching the NHL and NBA playoffs simultaneously.

"Listen to this," I said.

I took his grunt as assent.

"This book says that if you have large breasts, you should try putting a rolled up pair of socks under the boob the baby is feeding on."

Another grunt.

"I think mine qualify as large."

A third grunt. I was getting somewhere.

"We need to buy some tube socks."

Nothing.

I continued. "Some tube socks that would fit Shaq."

"What did you say about Shaq? Neither he nor the Lakers are having a great game."

"I don't care, but I need his size socks. You know, for my Shaq-sized boobs."

"You need socks for your boobs?"

"Weren't you listening?" I asked.

"Yes. I mean not really. I kind of zoned out to my own world when you mentioned your knockers."

"The book says I need to put socks under my boobs while I breastfeed. I have basketball breasts, so I need Shaq socks."

"What book?" he asked.

"The one I'm reading."

"Right," Chris said. "Do your breasts need anything else?"

I finally had his attention.

"Look," I said, distracting him, "halftime's over. What's the score?"

In those last weeks of pregnancy, sleep was as elusive as an Oscar nomination for the average reality TV star. I started a sleep debt that I'd spend the next ten years trying to recover from. Often I woke up and read. I was on Pregnancy Book #83.

Some nights my hip went numb. Some nights I'd urinate hourly. Some nights I'd be karate kicked in the ribs by a fetal black belt.

I emailed my pregnant cousin: "Lefty has taken up the pommel horse. This is likely the only time either of my kids will be small enough to contemplate gymnastics."

I waxed on about stats and bodily functions, and I pressed send.

I found Chris watching sports again—this time hockey playoffs—escaping into a world where the season didn't last for the rest of his life.

"We need to preregister our kids for speed skating," I said.

"We need to *what*?"

"Preregister them for speed skating," I explained. "With our genes, each babe is bound to be a head on thunder thighs."

Chris smiled. "Short track cycling is an option too."

"True," I said. "And it has a complementary off season."

We laughed.

"Speaking of compliments, I could use one," I said.

His smile grew. "You look good knocked up."

 Parenting Tip: Before placing your children in sports activities, consider their genetic limitations. Blame your spouse for any shortfalls.

Hard as those hot, smelly months may have been, they weren't as difficult as other people's verbal blunders. Friends, colleagues, and relatives, perhaps well meaning, trespassed into what was, in pre-pregnant days, forbidden territory: commenting on my weight, mood, and appearance.

It started in my first trimester, when I was two months pregnant and on modified bed rest. An acquaintance visited me and shared that she had miscarried twins three times. *Thanks*, I thought, *I'll sleep way more soundly now.*

When I was back at work in my second trimester, I attempted to resolve a minor conflict with a colleague. He said, "Do you think you're being oversensitive because you're pregnant?"

No, I thought, *I'm being oversensitive because you're an idiot with a teaching degree.*

When I was seven months pregnant, I arrived at a party wearing a funky T-shirt with a wild print. A single woman came up to me with her martini and said, "It's hard to get nice maternity clothes, isn't it?"

I'd like you shaken, not stirred, I thought.

One month later, I was an inflatable oven lacking an off switch. I visited with a woman in the supermarket line, who announced, "Oh my God, you're *so* small for being eight months pregnant."

Finally, I made it to month nine. I put out an APB for my ankles, which had been missing for a few weeks. As I watched a school baseball game, my colleague's brother said, "You look like you're carrying a *really big* baby."

Parenting Tip: Record all the stupid things people say to you while pregnant. Stop after you give birth; you won't have enough free time to jot down the stupid things people say to parents.

After hearing the last of these comments, I waddled home and whined. I sat under that lone ceiling fan once again, put up my feet, and looked at that-body-part-formerly-known-as-my-ankles. Chris brought me yet another glass of water, condensation already dripping, and a paper towel to catch the falling droplets.

"Why do so many people say stupid things to pregnant women?" I asked.

Chris sat down beside me. "Do you think they're jealous?" he said.

"Of this?" I pointed to my belly, which may have contained Goliath's offspring.

"Yes," he said, patting my belly in deep appreciation, "of this."

"Maybe," I said, guzzling the water, wishing it were a beer.

"At least it only lasts nine months," he added.

"True," I said, wiping my forehead with the paper towel. "This means we're a week or two away from people starting to criticize how we're raising our kids."

CAN YOU IMAGINE IF TARANTINO MADE A FILM ABOUT PREGNANCY AND BIRTH?

On the Monday before our twins were born, we met with our doctor for the last time. We knew he'd set a date for the delivery; we'd just assumed it'd be the following week. Somehow "next week" had very different psychological ramifications than "this Saturday," the date he gave us. Moments after the appointment, we walked towards the pharmacy. My pulse raced and I understood why people have babies in hospitals: because it's highly likely the adults will pass out at some point. We held hands and spoke in jumbled thoughts.

"This Satur—"

"I know. I can't even—"

"—day. That's not even next—"

"—imagine that. I have so much—"

"—week. It's this week. Do you think—"

"—to do. Mom and Patti fly—"

"—we're ready to be parents? I guess we—"

"—in Saturday night. Can you pick—"

"—don't have a choice."

"—them up?"

As we waited for the pharmacist to fill my last prescription of Ventolin tablets, the anti-contraction medicine I'd been on for ten weeks, we replayed our conversation. Chris assured me that he'd meet my mom and sister at the airport Saturday night, a dozen hours after the scheduled birth of our insta-family.

Then we went to preregister for our hospital stay.

"What package do you want?" the woman asked.

Package?

Our choices were the three-night/two-nurse option that included doctors' fees for 32,000 Baht ($1,040), or the four-night/four-nurse option that did not include doctors' fees for 38,000 Baht ($1,235). Of course, there would be "an additional surcharge for the extra baby."

It was more than a bit surreal, like checking into a four-star hotel on Jupiter. I wanted to ask if I could book a facial or if they took frequent flyer miles.

"So," the woman said, "how many nurses would you like?"

"How many nurses?" I repeated. "I'd like one more than I'll need."

She smiled, lips pursed like she was expelling gas. "We don't have that option."

"I don't think I'm qualified to make this decision," I said. "Shouldn't someone who has a medical degree be making it?"

She smiled again.

"How much does our insurance cover?" Chris asked.

I glared at him as only a very pregnant woman could. "Just put us down for a fleet of nurses," I said.

"Feet?" the Thai woman said. "I'm sorry, I do not know what 'feet of nurses' means."

"Just a lot. I'm going to need a lot of nurses."

"Of course you will," she said, noting something on my registration form, likely "Psych Consult Recommended."

Later at home, the pace continued. Chris was maniacally opening and shutting DVD cases.

"Can you please stop what you're doing?" I asked.

"Sorry," he said. "I have to get this done."

I watched him reorder DVDs on our bookshelf.

"Are you alphabetizing them?" I asked.

"Maybe?" he said, half embarrassed.

"Come sit down," I said.

He flopped next to me and playfully whacked my thigh with *Pulp Fiction*.

"You know," I continued, "the babies won't care if your DVDs are alphabetized."

"True," he said, "but it's one thing I can do where I can see the result."

I nodded.

"Do you want some help? I'm pretty good with A to G, thanks to fluctuations in my bra size."

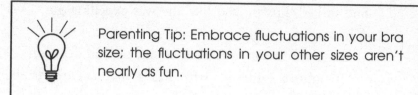

Parenting Tip: Embrace fluctuations in your bra size; the fluctuations in your other sizes aren't nearly as fun.

"I think I'm OK," he said.

"Can you imagine if Tarantino made a film about pregnancy and birth?" I said.

Chris laughed. "I think that would be the start of the end of the human race."

THE SAPPY FILES, PART 1 (OR WHY MY KIDS' FUTURE THERAPISTS SHOULD BE KIND)

Dear Babies,

It's just over twelve hours until the scheduled C-section. You're going to be born on May 29 around 8:00 AM. That's twelve hours from now, not even a blink in the universe's concept of time.

I don't really know what to say to you, so I'm going to tell you about this week.

Your dad seems to have gone into overdrive, with anticipatory stress invading his body. His jerky movements and inability to focus make him seem like he's had sudden onset ADHD. He's a gamer, however, and will be a star tomorrow. I hope I will be too.

But the real stars are you two. I don't yet know if you're both boys or if you're both girls or if you're one of each. Regardless, you two are loved, not just by us, but by a bevy of people. Your birth is almost an event. People are genuinely ecstatic for us. We've had sincere offers from people to drive us places, to cook for us, to play tour guide for your grandma and auntie when they arrive, to sit with us. Today, we've had phone calls from Jerusalem and Singapore, and your dad received so many handshakes, good wishes, and free food at work that he's probably contracted (or ingested) some tropical virus.

You are community babies, in many ways. People who I didn't even think were religious are praying for your safe arrival. I feel that we are so blessed already and you two are loved beyond measure before anyone has met you.

Last night, our second last night alone, I had a few tears as I looked at your dad and said, "I have no idea what I'm doing."

He replied, "Neither do I, but between the two of us we have over seventy years of life experience, so I'm hoping we can figure things out." It's odd having children when you're older and established in your career. You're so used to being competent and experienced that it's disconcerting to be a novice again, especially in this, the most important job we have. I hope we don't mess it up. I hope I don't mess you up.

I'm going to miss your kicking contests, the silent companionship, but I know I need to let go of this stage to get to the next one. Perhaps that's the big lesson of parenthood, or even of life: You need to let go and trust in the next stage, not holding (your kids or yourself) back.

I'm ready to meet you.

Goodbye pregnancy books; hello baby books. And babies. Yes. Hello, babies.

Love,

Mommy? Mom? Mama? Crazy Pregnant Lady?

PART TWO

THE FIRST TWELVE MONTHS, OR THE I-BARELY-REMEMBER YEAR

PLEASE TAKE THESE CRYING THINGS AWAY

We were in the operating room. It was 7:55 AM. The epidural headache had come and gone. Chris stood beside me, holding my hand. So far, everything was going according to my Caesarean Birth Plan, which was the length of a PhD thesis. The room was cold, bright, sterile, busy. A short blue drape sat on my boobs so I couldn't see the doctors. They were joking in Thai.

There are many things I love about the Thais, and one is that they love to have fun when they work. One anesthetist, two obstetricians, two pediatricians, and four nurses—more than I ordered—fluttered about, laughing.

Before I could say, *Did you cut off my legs because I can't feel them*, it became quiet. Dr. K, our ob-gyn guy, looked down and soon the other medical personnel took his direction and began the business of their morning: slicing open my uterus with a razor-sharp scalpel.

I can't remember if time passed quickly or slowly.

At 8:00 AM, I heard a cry and saw Dr. K hold up a gray, goopy alien. "Your first child," he announced, "is a boy."

I started crying. Might as well join my son.

A nurse held him up to my face for a brief cuddle and then took him away for de-goop-ification. My stare turned to the doctors' faces again. Dr. K appeared to be kneading my womb with his elbow or forearm.

I glanced at Chris, whose mouth was agape. I remember thinking, *This might be the part when husbands pass out.*

"Is he doing a wrestling maneuver on my uterus?" I asked.

Chris rose—his posture and expression morphing to Supreme Alpha Male, his eyes flitting from Dr. K to my womb.

One of the doctor's sidekicks looked at us. "Go," he ordered Chris. "Be with your son." He gestured to the goop-off station. Chris backed down and staggered to a crying boy.

At 8:02 AM, a seeming eternity later, Dr. K held up the second of my litter. "Your second child," he declared, "is a girl."

A nurse brought her to me. I cuddled my goopy girl and sobbed. Chris joined me in tears and in closeness, cradling our slightly-less-goopy boy.

After our babies were de-gooped and baked in incubators, we were reunited in our standard room, complete with fridge, balcony, and two babies. I tossed my breast near one of the babies' mouths, seeing if I were indeed a mammal. Chris, meanwhile, hovered over our other baby, holding up a diaper the size of a cigarette package.

A nurse in starched uniform and hat breezed in, clipboard in hand. I hoped she wasn't grading us on technique.

"What are the babies' names?" she asked.

"The girl's first name is Vivian," I said.

"And how do you spell Vivian?" she asked.

"V-I-V-I—" I stopped. I looked at Chris. "I don't know how to spell their names. I never thought about it. Did you?"

"Not really," he said, putting down the diaper and covering the boy with a blanket.

The nurse scrawled something on her clipboard. Likely an F, for *Freaking*. As in freaking horrible parents.

"How about V-I-V-I-A-N?" I said to Chris.

"Sounds good to me."

The nurse repeated the spelling. I nodded.

William's name was slightly more straightforward.

 Parenting Tip: Discuss the spelling of your baby's name before an official lady with a clipboard corners you.

"We will have the birth certificate for you shortly," the nurse said.

I fazed out, focusing on how not to breastfeed.

"Is it in English?" Chris asked.

The nurse smiled. "It's in Thai."

"In Thai script?" Chris asked. We barely knew how to order beer in Thai; we certainly couldn't read or write the curly-cue script.

"Yes," she smiled.

"Can we get one in English?" Chris said.

"*Mai pen rai*. You just have to go to an official translator."

"Well, I'm glad it's no problem," Chris said. "How do we find one of those?"

"Someone else will tell you," she smiled. "*Mai pen rai*."

She sailed out, clipboard in hand.

Chris shrugged, and I went back to playing "Where's the Nipple: the newborn's Waldo-esque quest."

Part of my post-birth plan included the following: Don't let the babies out of my sight. Ever. When the doctors removed my placentas, I'm pretty sure the part of my brain that reasons went too. I threw out psychotic mommy questions with the frequency of a pitcher warming up in the bullpen: What if someone took one of our babies? What if someone took the other one of our babies? What if the nurses snuck formula into them to shut them up? What if the nurses couldn't shut them up? What if I couldn't recognize them in the nursery amid all the other wrinkly blobs?

So, I did what any overwhelmed, immobile new mother would do: I became Stalker Mom, vowing never to let my spawn out of my sight.

This worked exceptionally well. For the first hour. And then the Law of Diminishing Returns went into effect.

"Are you sure you don't want us to take them to the nursery?" the nurses asked.

"They're fine here."

It didn't matter that I couldn't get out of bed with my Caesarean gash or that I had no clue how to breastfeed two babies, with or without tube socks.

After hour twenty-two without sleep, I told Chris, nearly asleep on the adjacent cot, "I have to get these babies out of here."

He mumbled something. It might have been, "This bed sucks," or "Shut those babies up."

I took it as assent and dialed the hospital's version of 9-1-1.

"Can you take my babies away?"

"Pardon me?"

"Please take these crying things away. Now."

"Is everything OK?"

"I wouldn't be calling if everything were OK. I need sleep."

"A nurse will be there in a moment."

I didn't hear a Code Red announcement, but I'm pretty sure maternity wards have another code for mommy-is-losing-it, remove-babies-at-once.

Before more urine could dribble into my catheter, two nurses rushed in. They each wheeled out six-plus pounds of baby.

I slept. Mercifully.

Parenting Tip: Take full advantage of the hospital's nursery while in the maternity ward. Those nurses aren't going to be around to help out when the kid is three years old.

FOLLOW THAT CAR. MY BABIES ARE IN THERE

I had been warned about lack of sleep and sore nipples and nonstop crying, but no one told me about peeing. Once Vivian and William were ripped from my abdomen, urinating became, well, impossible.

I had been catheterized. That little instrument-of-terror didn't come out until the next day, the same day my urethra curled up and went into Al Qaeda–like hiding.

I already felt like I couldn't walk or breastfeed or sleep for more than two hours. Now, in my de-catheterized state, I couldn't even pee.

A Type-A nurse gave me and my full bladder a how-to lesson on urinating.

I sat on the toilet. She turned on the cold-water faucet. "Think of a waterfall," she said. "You hear the water falling a long way—"

"Can I jump?" I asked.

"Pardon me?"

"Never mind."

I shifted on the toilet seat, stretching to turn the tap off.

"Leave the water on," she instructed.

Water shortage be damned, I left it on.

"Just try. And relax."

She walked out. And I cried my own waterfall, tears that morphed into sobs. If you can curl up into a fetal position while sitting on a toilet, I did just that.

Chris heard the commotion.

"You OK in there?"

"What kind of human being can't even pee?" I yelled over the sound of the water.

He came to the door. "Umm . . . the kind that miraculously birthed two healthy babies yesterday?"

I sobbed louder as Bangkok's canals filled with the sink's water.

"I can't do anything right."

Great. A heart-to-heart on the toilet. Chris opened the door.

I continued. "If I can't pee, how can I possibly be a mom?"

The nurse came back in. There were now two people watching me fail to urinate.

"You're doing just fine," she said.

"But I can't even pee," I said.

"You will. I promise." She assisted me and my full bladder back to bed.

One hour later, there was a slow leak in the dam. My urethra uncurled, and I peed.

I flushed the toilet, washed my hands, and emerged from the bathroom to hear Chris singing the Hallelujah Chorus. I laughed, my first one in forty-eight hours.

 Parenting Tip: Celebrate small postpartum miracles, like being able to pee and poo. Mourn the big realities, like having to leave the hospital with your baby.

Now that I could successfully pee and poo, I was deemed competent.

"You're doing great," Dr. K said on Day Three. "Your milk has come in. Your babies are healthy. You can go home tomorrow."

"What? Tomorrow? You can't send me home with these babies. Not by myself."

"You're all by yourself?"

"Well, not really," I said. "My mom and sister are here from Canada. And my husband. But . . . I mean . . . without nurses at night."

He sensed my panic and smiled. "You can stay longer if you like."

I had become used to my private room with a nurse available at the push of a button. Every night since the first endless one, I'd called the nurses' station at nine o'clock, and they'd come to cart my twins to the nursery. Florence Nightingale would call me when my spawn needed to be fed and I'd walk the green mile. I wasn't executed, though breastfeeding occasionally made me wish for it; still, I persevered because I'm a mammal and because I had two nurses as my handmaidens—more support than I could've wished for.

"So, I can stay longer?" I asked my doctor.

"Yes."

"How does two more days sound?" I suggested, forgetting that I didn't have a medical degree.

"Fine."

To celebrate, I called Starbucks and they delivered a Mango Frappuccino to my room. It helped me pee.

In addition to enjoying swanky room-delivered beverages, I sampled udon and miso soup from the hospital's Japanese restaurant, which seemed pleased to serve me in my pajamas.

I loved the Bangkok hospital's rooftop garden and my in-room fridge filled with calories, but some of the country's practices seemed a bit, well, foreign. When the staff got my twins ready to send home, nurses swaddled them in blankets and knotted the ends by their toes. Vivian and William looked like cute caterpillars, but their cocoons weren't exactly conducive to using car seats, which were not the norm in Thailand. Good luck finding any seatbelts in a *tuk tuk*, let alone on the back of a motorcycle taxi or in a cab.

After the nurses bundled William and Vivian for their journey home, they put them in clear Rubbermaid bassinets. "We can just carry them down to the lobby," I said.

"Sorry," one nurse said. "Hospital policy."

Then she took out the Costco-sized box of plastic wrap. I watched in amazement.

She smiled at me and said, "Hospital policy when we transport them floor to floor."

At this point I called Chris, who was taking care of the hospital bill, which included the six-nurse package. "The nurse just covered our twins in Saran Wrap."

"She what?"

"She covered their bassinet things with plastic wrap. Their heads aren't covered, so I'm pretty sure they can breathe."

"I'll be right there."

We survived the treacherous trip in the elevator. Vivian and William were not inclined to test the plastic-wrap-roll-bar and neither were we.

We had enough *Amazing Race* roadblocks ahead of us.

Moments later, I endured another sob-fest. This time, I stood outside of Starbucks in the hospital lobby. Chris was calling the driver he'd hired so we could actually seatbelt our babes in for the five-minute ride home, which featured crossing the world's most dangerous, uncontrolled road. Each time I crossed that intersection in a cab while pregnant, I curled up on the backseat, closed my eyes, and hummed "Jesus Loves Me," a technique that had helped me survive driving in India years before.

There I was, latte-less, and sobbing again. My mom rubbed my back. My sister tried to talk to me.

"I can't go home with my babies," I wailed.

"What do you mean?" my sister asked.

"There's not enough room. Chris is going to go with them. I'm not allowed to lift them when they're in their car seats."

My Caesarean gash was still raw and my internal organs had been pushed around when the doctor did his wrestling move on my uterus.

"We'll just get a cab and follow them," my sister said.

I sucked up my tears and watched my sister—an experienced and calm mom of two—show Chris how to attach and secure the car seats.

The hospital's bellboy hailed a cab. We got in. I gave the address in Thai. We followed Chris and the babies.

My crying fit was under control—until we got to death-trap road, just 300 feet from the hospital's doors. Crossing this street was like playing chicken in the Indy 500, blindfolded. To get across the five-lane road, the taxi driver had to nose the car out, one lane at a time, and pray that Buddha-on-the-dashboard was having a good day. Do this successfully through four more lanes, and reincarnation was delayed. Building a hospital beside this intersection was a sound business investment.

I watched Chris and the babies edge through lane one. I cried, closed my eyes, and hummed Sunday school songs at a frantic tempo. Then our taxi driver turned right.

I opened my eyes. "Go straight," I shouted in Thai.

The driver replied that he couldn't. It wasn't safe.

"Follow that car," I said. "My babies are in there."

He looked at me. "*Maidai.*"

"What do you mean you *can't*? Of course you can. The other car went straight."

By now, it was too late. My babies had made it across the deathtrap and we were going the long way. I could almost feel the remains of my imaginary umbilical cord being torn.

And I'd lost my temper. In Thai culture, public outrage is looked down upon because everyone who witnessed the outburst loses. Defeated, I called Chris and sobbed. Again.

Five minutes later, the taxi pulled up to our apartment building. I crawled out and apologized to the driver for my nervous breakdown while Chris paid him a week's wages in compensation. My mom hugged me and I looked at my two little post-goop balls.

They'd slept the entire ride home.

CAN YOU STOP SELLING BOOB-SHOW PASSES TO OUR GUESTS?

After they changed 200 diapers in ten days, my mom and sister left the country. Round one of my mastitis meds kicked in. Vivian and William slept. Kind of.

Chris and I sat in our Bangkok living room enjoying the silence amid sweltering heat, the kind that requires the Jaws of Life to unstick your thighs from each other. We waited, like soldiers in the jungle, our senses alert to any change in our immediate environment. I watched the ceiling fan slice at the humidity, until a newborn cry—a stark screech—shattered the moment. We jumped, startled by our own artillery fire. Crap.

It was now only weeks into our biggest job, parenting twins, and neither Chris nor I had any experience that mattered. With four and a half university degrees between us, you would think we could figure out what was wrong with our progeny, two little squirts whose age was still measured in weeks. I mean, we could quote Shakespeare at length and tell you how the Library of Congress catalog system was organized (two facts that explained why dinner party invitations were scarce), but we couldn't tell you why our kids cried. Plus, now that my mom and sister had returned to Canada, we were alone with these mewling, puking things.

I can't remember what I did to stop the wailing; perhaps I changed a diaper, removed a blanket, or stood on my head for the length of *King Lear*.

When I emerged from the bowels of the bedroom, Chris asked, "Who was crying?"

"Who was crying?" I repeated. "Well, one of the babies." Sarcasm had become my postpartum specialty.

"I know that," he answered. "Which one?"

"Oh, it was, uh . . . I think . . ." I wracked my short-term memory, which since having children had become the length of a text message. "It was what's-his-name . . . the guy."

Parenting Tip: Strive to remember the name of your baby. Write it on your hand if you have to. Remembering your spouse's name is optional.

"You mean *William?*" Chris asked. His neurons were firing faster than mine, possibly because he hadn't spawned two babies and two placentas.

"Um, yes, William."

I sat down again, stared at the ceiling fan, and waited for the other one, what's-her-name.

The wait wasn't long. More shrill cries pierced the air, not counting mine. Chris and I stared at each other with the intensity of Uri Geller willing a spoon to bend, each silently bidding the other do something about the noise. A conversation ensued.

"Someone's crying."

"Yep."

"Which one?"

"The girl."

"You sure?"

"Not really."

"Why's she crying?"

"I dunno."

"Any ideas?"

"Nothing concrete."

"Is she wet?"

"Nope."

"Hungry?"

"Don't think so."

"Tired?"

"Beats me."

"Hot? . . . Cold?"

"Normal a few minutes ago."

"So, you don't know why she's crying?"

"No. You?"

"Nope."

"I understand why some people beat their kids."

"You what?"

"Seriously. We're educated, older, financially secure, happy enough in our mar—"

"Happy enough?"

"You know what I mean."

"I do?"

"Yes. And sometimes we still feel like dangling them over the balcony."

"Like Michael Jackson."

"Only we'd never do it."

"Yeah, we're too hot to move from this couch unless the guy or what's-her-name screams bloody murder."

Of course we eventually moved . . . to our bedroom. We were starting to mimic Vivian and William's cycle of cry, eat, poop, sleep.

On occasion Vivian and William managed to sleep at the same time. There's something peaceful about sleeping babies. Unless you think they're dead.

One night, Chris and I stood over them and watched our two angels asleep in the same crib, feeling like the world's best parents—or at least better than a tortoise who has dumped her eggs in a hole and swam off into the ocean. We smiled at the perfect moment.

Until I said, "They're not dead, are they?"

"I don't think so," Chris answered. He looked at me. "Do you think they're dead?"

We hovered over the crib like two novice marine biologists inspecting a polluted aquarium for signs of life. "I can't see them breathing," I said.

"You can't see me breathe either."

"Point for you."

"Do you think we should wake them up?" Chris asked.

"No. You never wake a sleeping baby. Waking two is criminal."

"What should we do then?"

"Let's jiggle them," I said.

"Jiggle? You want to jiggle them?"

"Don't look at me like I'm about to pick them up and Shake n' Bake them. I'm just talking about jiggling."

"Jiggling? What does that mean?"

I defined the word. "I'll just put my hand on one of their backs and wiggle it to see if they move."

"That's wiggling, not jiggling," he said.

"Thanks, Webster."

I placed my hand on each baby's back and jiggle-wiggled. They both moved.

"They're not dead."

"Not dead at all."

"Do you think this qualifies me to guest star on *CSI*?" I asked.

"Not likely." He kissed me on my forehead. "Maybe Animal Planet."

Parenting Tip: If you fear your sleeping baby is dead, jiggle-wiggle her.

Night never lasted long enough. On the odd occasion we managed to sleep simultaneously, William and Vivian's wake-up cries were like amplified foghorns.

For two cat-sized creatures, Vivian and William were loud, especially when they were hungry. Breastfeeding them gave me a close affinity to other mammals. With my wee litter camping out at my boobs, I couldn't help but remember that mangy barn cat that crept around my parents' farm, lying on her back while sharp-clawed kitties fought their way to her teats. Any mammal that sprawls on her back that much is in for a lot of trouble.

Because I didn't want to breastfeed every waking hour, I made Chris get up in the middle of the night to help me feed the kids. He hadn't learned to lactate, which would've been handy, but he could wipe butts and hand me clean babies so I could position their floppy heads onto a breastfeeding pillow bigger than Maui.

At first I tried the big-breast-sock-trick. I don't think putting rolled up socks under my boobs helped me breastfeed, but they did help me in another way: they were weapons. I hurled them at Chris whenever I was frustrated with "natural" breastfeeding, something women have been doing as long as men have been grunting.

"Thanks for not throwing a book," Chris said, retrieving the socks.

"This isn't natural, you know," I said.

"Chucking socks at your husband?"

"No. Breastfeeding two babies. At least it doesn't feel natural."

"Do you want to try just one baby at a time?" he asked.

"No way," I said. "I already nurse them close to eight hours a day. If I do sixteen, I'm sending them back."

"I don't think there's a return policy."

I yawned. "I didn't read the fine print." I inhaled deeply and looked down at our babies. After having a bit of milk, they'd both fallen asleep, little sunbathers on my island cushion. I repositioned the guy under my right arm, woke him by jiggle-wiggling, and shoved my right breast in his mouth. I repeated with what's-her-name.

Parenting Tip: Read the fine print and the non-existent return policy *before* you get knocked up.

"You know what they call this?" I asked.

"I'd say *breastfeeding*?" Chris answered.

I launched another pair of socks at him. "The way I'm holding them," I said. "Do you know what it's called?"

"I've got no idea."

"A football hold."

"Really?"

"Yup," I said. "According to one of the books at least. They're tucked under my arms like footballs."

Chris smiled. "Are you going to run them in for a touchdown?"

"Pretty sure there'd be a flag on the play. Given that I'm carrying two balls."

"I carry two balls," Chris said.

I laughed, startling both babies. One of my spawn lost suction, and a freed breast sent a continuous stream of milk into the air and across the room.

"It's the halftime show," Chris said.

I fought to control the leak, dousing a baby and a nearby wall with milk. "Now stop making me laugh," I said. "I've got to connect to my inner mammal."

"OK. But if you feel like kicking them for a field goal, let me know.

"Will do," I said. "This one needs changing."

"William?"

"Yes, the guy."

Parenting Tip: Nighttime breastfeeding sessions are more entertaining if you wake your spouse. Just tell him he's *bonding* with his child.

Now it was time for my middle-of-the-night entertainment: watching Chris change the other twin's diaper. When William lay on the changing table, I was reminded of the Fountains of Bellagio. I could watch this nightly; sometimes I did. As soon as the dirty diaper was off, the show started. Will's back arched and his penis extended, unleashing a perfect stream of urine in Chris's face.

Vivian's specialty was impeccably timed green diarrhea. I'm not sure how an innocent baby can empty her bowels a nanosecond after you lay her on the change table, remove her soggy diaper, and raise her legs to clean her bum. But as soon as Chris reached this stage with Vivian, a jet of hot liquid poo sprayed from her butt to his black pajamas, turning him into a canvas.

"That crap on your shirt looks like a Jackson Pollock painting," I said.

"Not funny," Chris answered, handing me clean Vivian.

It may not have been art, but it was solid—or at least semi-solid—entertainment at 3:00 AM.

The gong show continued whenever guests popped over, a frequent occurrence in our close-knit expatriate community. When the doorbell rang, Chris warned our visitors that they were going to get a free boob display and to enter only if they were unfazed, because once feeding time came, modesty disappeared.

But this was Bangkok; people could see ping-pong and goldfish girlie shows four blocks away. Don't ask. Unless you "wanna make boom-boom long time!"

Later, Chris seemed to catch on to the fact that he could be making money off me.

"Ten bucks a boob or fifteen for a double pass," he joked at the door.

"Seriously?" I said after that round of visitors had left. "Can you stop selling boob-show passes to our guests?" I tried to suppress a smile.

He grinned. Then he said the same line the next time our doorbell rang, making me laugh yet again.

DO YOU THINK THEY DROPPED OUR BABIES INTO A BIG VAT OF SOUP?

According to Thai law, one parent has to have an un-pronounceable surname of 39.3 letters (like Prisan-iripiyanporniratpattanasai) in order to get a Thai passport. According to Canadian law, expatriate parents need to fill out more forms than an accountant does in April in order for their children to be granted Canadian citizenship. I'm pretty sure the Wikipedia entry for "Canadian Pastimes" reads: "Waiting behind Plexiglas, be it at a hockey game or an embassy in Thailand."

To satisfy one of the Canadian government's require-ments, we needed passport pictures of our newborns. William and Vivian's virgin outing, therefore, was to a photo studio.

After figuring out how the Baby Bjorn carriers worked—an activity that made assembling an IKEA desk with your teeth look easy—Chris and I set out, each with a two-week-old heat pack Velcro-ed to our chest. We walked for ten minutes, past a seamstress, motorbike taxi drivers, and the papaya lady before arriving at Sukhumvit Road, one of Bangkok's busiest thoroughfares. We climbed the stairs to a photo studio, handed over the embassy's book of instructions, and began the challenge of unbinding two sweaty, floppy-necked babies without dropping them.

The photographer opened the instructions on the counter. "The background needs to be white," he read. "Can you place them here?" He pointed to a white screen nailed four feet up on the wall.

"No," I said. "They're not that tall."

"Can you just hold them up with your hands out of the picture?"

"No. They can't exactly hold up their heads." Pointing out the obvious had become *my* pastime.

He paused, looking around the scantly furnished room. "We will put the baby on this chair. I'll look for something white to cover it with."

I looked at the blue armless desk chair complete with casters.

"Isn't there anything else?" Chris asked.

By now, sweat rolled off all four of us. The slow ceiling fan mocked me.

"We could try this," the man said. He held up a gray towel that looked like it hadn't seen a washing machine since the Duggars were childless.

"Hold her," I said, placing Vivian in Chris's free arm. I took off my white shirt and put it on the chair, grateful that I had worn a tank top underneath. I fussed with the shirt, trying to get it wrinkle free. After I locked the chair's wheels into place, I took sleeping Vivian and laid her on my shirt. I sat on the floor near the casters, at first spotting her like she was a gymnast on a trampoline, then propping her up like a doll when she began to slide to the edge. I ducked as the photographer got ready to take her picture.

He looked through the shutter, paused, and pulled back. "She needs to open her eyes. It's regulation."

"You want a two-week-old to open her eyes on command? Are you serious?" I asked from my spot on the floor.

He nodded toward the counter. "The instructions."

"I didn't think they came with instructions," I mumbled.

Chris said something back that sounded like a cross between air escaping a tire and a Welsh curse.

> Parenting Tip: Shipping your baby via FedEx or DHL is easier than getting a passport photo with your baby's eyes open.

I picked up what's-her-name, pulled out a wet wipe intended for a diaper change, and cleaned her face. Her eyes blinked open, then closed. I sighed. Chris shifted; Supreme Alpha Male was ready to erupt. The photographer smiled and bowed slightly.

I pulled out my water bottle, doused the cloth, and squeezed it on Vivian's face. She started to wail. I ducked back under the chair, held her waist, and listened for the shutter.

"We got one," the photographer said.

"Freaking Hallelujah," Chris said as we switched babies. "And now for William."

I looked at William; he was sweaty and sleeping.

My eyes shifted to the wet wipes, then to my water bottle. No contest.

Like a player who's just won the Super Bowl, I picked up my water bottle and dumped it over the baldish head of the one who calls the shots.

Our little coach woke up. We got the championship photo.

Eventually, I began to venture out myself. We'd hired a nanny/housemaid to help me for six hours each weekday. With our closest family member 8,000 miles away, it was either hire Mary Poppins or put the babies on a bamboo raft down the Chao Phraya River and hope the daughter of the King of Siam would find them among the sewage.

When I left our apartment, I would often take one baby—usually in a Baby Bjorn carrier so I wouldn't have to maneuver the limo-sized double stroller. Our nanny would take the other twin with her on errands. Divide and conquer.

On one particular errand day, I took William. After walking past competing tailors who were trying to convince me I needed better clothes, I headed towards the mini-supermarket to pick up ice cream. I was a ball of sweat because carrying fourteen pounds through carbon dioxide emissions when it's ninety-eight degrees out will do that to you. I trudged up to the door and saw the sweaty Coca-Cola deliveryman holding Vivian. Our nanny was nowhere in sight.

"Hi," I said. "You're holding my baby." I thought of what one of the books said about germs and babies.

"Wiwian is your baby?" he asked, smiling and rocking Vivian. Thais have trouble saying Vs and Ls, whereas I have trouble saying all of the Thai consonants.

Before I could answer, the deliveryman shifted Vivian into his other arm and reached out to tickle William's toes, which stuck out of the baby carrier I wore. "And this is Wee-yum," he said, assuring me he knew my son's name. William giggled when the man tickled him again.

"OK, then," I said, "we're just going into the store."

I walked into the store with William and saw our nanny paying for some items we needed, like diapers, vodka, and Xanax. We chatted until one of the cashiers squealed over William, called him by name, and took him out of the carrier so I could shop unrestricted in cooler temperatures.

I beelined to the ice cream section and opened the cooler, the concrete jungle's instant air-conditioning.

I paid for my Häagen-Dazs (some habits didn't end with pregnancy), took William, and met my nanny outside. She held Vivian and the shopping bags. The Coca-Cola deliveryman had fled the scene. We walked home with our loads.

> Parenting Tip: Keep your household well stocked with these items essential to newborns: diapers, wipes, alcohol, alcohol, and alcohol.

Chris was back from work when we entered our apartment. Our nanny gave Vivian to him, unpacked our groceries, and prepared to depart.

I deposited William into his bouncy chair and unwrapped my ice cream. "I saw the Coca-Cola deliveryman holding one of our babies," I said.

"Really? Two days ago, I saw one of the hair stylists holding William."

"What's that saying about a village?" I asked, digging into my ice cream.

"It takes a village to raise a child."

"Well," I said, licking some chocolate off my lips, "we don't need a village. Only a nanny and a few retailers."

And some waitresses, as we would soon find out.

Later that week, after I was sick of the bare walls of our apartment, Chris and I decided to take Vivian and William out for dinner to a place we called The Concrete Slab. The size of an NFL field, the Slab was adorned with cheap plastic patio furniture in various shades of dirty white. Several portable propane cooking stations lined the outside. Megaphone-style speakers distorted Thai music. It may have been romantic if you were inebriated and child-free.

Our pregnant friend accompanied us, her husband out of town. Chris left for the Slab's sidelines to order each of our favorite dishes: spicy pork, fried rice noodles, and chicken fried rice. I rocked the stroller with my foot and focused on having an adult conversation while not falling off the chair, a wobbly piece that seemed to have shrunk since I gave birth.

Before long, four Thai workers who looked vaguely familiar came up. "Twins?" they asked. I nodded. "Can we hold them?"

I looked at Vivian and William who were starting to squirm. "Sure."

The women unstrapped them from the stroller and cradled them. "We go for a walk?"

I shrugged. "Sure."

When Chris came back with our fried goodness, my friend and I were in the middle of the first conversation I'd had in weeks that didn't involve bodily fluids.

"I hate to interrupt," Chris said, placing our meals in front of us like he was a maitre d'. "Have either of you noticed that two babies are missing?"

"Four ladies took them for a walk," I said.

"OK . . ."

"Don't worry. I threw out that book."

"What book?" Chris asked.

"The one that said to protect your babies from strangers' germs. You know, after the Coke guy held Vivian."

"OK . . ."

"Don't worry. The women who took them work here." I looked around and saw plenty of women but none holding my DNA. "Uh oh. I can't see them." I checked the stroller to ensure it was empty. "Do you think they dropped our babies into a big vat of soup?"

"No," Chris said, digging into his spicy pork. "They don't sell soup here."

YOU SPIT AT THE TAXI DRIVERS WHILE PUSHING THE STROLLER?

We got our babies back. Then a few days later, Chris decided to take them for a stroll without attentive Thai waitresses or the Food Source (otherwise known as me).

While Chris was on his first solo outing with the twins, I was off to find nursing bras that fit so I could end my recurring mastitis.

Mastitis—the infection and inflammation of breast tissue—can be as painful as childbirth. In case men wish to imagine having mastitis, here is an analogy in three easy steps: (1) when you have a fever of 102°F, take a few Viagra tablets; (2) rub the juice from a hot pepper onto your penis; and (3) put on a pair of jeans three sizes too small and bash yourself in the crotch with a ball peen hammer.

Having recurring mastitis made me as pleasant as Gordon Ramsay locked in a meat cooler with Mike Tyson.

I knew it had something to do with wearing the wrong bra size. I could write a book on wearing the wrong bra size. Sometime during university, I got fitted for a bra and my life changed, or so I imagined. Add a decade, pregnancy, and breastfeeding twins, and I was heading further into the bra alphabet, to XXX territory.

I was in the wrong country.

I had been down this road before with footwear. Weeks after arriving in Bangkok, I realized that I could not purchase any size ten shoes for women. So, when I was in a beach town, I saw a posse of transvestites. I chased them down, stopped one who was taller (and had shapelier legs) than me, and asked him where he bought her shoes.

With bras, it wasn't quite as easy. Transvestites and transgenders tend not to have big racks. Thai women wear bras that come in battery sizes: AAA to C. You can occasionally find a D. Once, I even found an F cup in one department store.

There were my breasts, red, hot, and oozing out some foreign substance in a too tight F-cup bra. For the third time.

My quest—to find a bra that fit—was on.

I had done some serious investigation. Eventually, through black market connections, I had learned that staff from the Wacoal bra factory visited one of the department stores weekly to measure Dolly Parton impersonators for custom fitted bras.

I began my pilgrimage at the same time Chris went on his virgin outing with the twins. After waiting in the department store for two hours, dangerously close to the twins' feeding time, I was seen by the bra factory people.

"What kind of bra do you want?" the lady asked. "Strapless?"

I laughed. "No. One with straps that will hold up two overripe mangos."

She looked at me for clarification.

"I need a nursing bra that goes halfway through the alphabet," I said.

"A big one?"

I nodded.

"No problem," she said. "But minimum order is three."

"OK. How much?"

"2,800 Baht total."

I did the math: ninety dollars. "No problem."

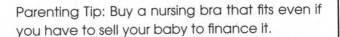 Parenting Tip: Buy a nursing bra that fits even if you have to sell your baby to finance it.

I walked into the change room, disrobed, and was measured in forty-seven places by a trio of Thai women. My breasts, meanwhile, knew it was time to feed my twins. So while the ladies measured and re-measured, milk dripped everywhere. I tried to think of anything but my babies: dead puppies, decomposing bats on power lines, even Leonardo DiCaprio falling off the *Titanic* during the opening credits, but my milk leaked, forming little pools on the floor amid my dignity.

"I'm sorry," I said, as one of the attendants got hit with milk.

The women giggled. "*Mai pen rai.*"

I smiled reluctantly. No problem, the Thai's beautiful answer to everything.

"When will the bras be ready?" I asked, stuffing my juicy mangos back into the too tight bra.

"Next Saturday," one of the women said, helping me fasten the clasp and adjust the straps of my boulder holder. "Is that OK?" she asked.

Mai pen rai.

When I got home, I stripped and fed my babies.

Chris, meanwhile, told me of his stroller escapades. His outing is one of those tales that becomes part of a family's lore. Due to my ooziness, I wasn't present, but somehow it's become my story too.

Not long after I left, Chris ferried William and Vivian down our building's refrigerator-sized elevator and deposited them into the limousine stroller, which was parked in the lobby since it didn't fit in the lift.

In the time our twins had been womb-less, Bangkok had not become more stroller—or wheelchair—accessible.

Chris did what was common if you were on a less-than-chaotic street: he pushed the stroller *on* the actual street, literally in the middle of the road.

He bypassed the mending woman set up with her vintage sewing machine and the blind man selling lottery tickets, pinging his way around with his rebar cane. It was midafternoon, which meant—like most other times of the day—the sun was relentless and the air was heavy. The mere act of being alive caused people to perspire; if they happened to be doing the push-the-twins-in-a-stroller obstacle course, a full-scale tourist sweat was guaranteed. Add a large man like Chris to this mix and you have rivers of perspiration.

Chris dodged another muffler-less *tuk tuk* before turning the corner, a feat as easy as steering an overloaded supermarket cart with a locked wheel across a rice paddy. Chris's shirt stuck to his back, he squinted in the sun, and he tried to ignore the jingle of the ice cream bike that was never quite out of hearing distance.

He neared the motorcycle taxi drivers. On this corner, there were always a dozen or more, a rough-looking bunch outfitted in matching vests, joking, playing the odd game of checkers with bottle caps, entertaining each other while waiting for customers.

With full smiles, they watched as Chris heaved the twins past them. They looked at the stroller and chatted to each other in Thai.

Then, as Chris trudged further along, one said, "Hey, *farang*. F-fat!"

Chris paused. He knew *farang* meant foreigner. And he was sick of the fat jokes.

"Yeah," chimed another, "f-fat!"

Chris stopped, wiped sweat off his forehead, and looked back. "What did you say?"

"F-fat!" one repeated, pointing at Chris and laughing with his buddies.

Chris unleashed a barrage of obscenities, held up his fists, and motioned "you wanna go?" before spitting on the ground and taking a shortcut home.

When Chris first told me this, I stopped him there. "You spit at the taxi drivers?" I said. "While pushing the stroller?"

I had been in Bangkok long enough to know that motor-cycle taxi guys knew where to hire a hit man for $100.

 Parenting Tip: Pray that no one puts a hit on your husband after he takes your newborn(s) on his first solo outing.

Later that day, we shared the story with a Thai friend who'd come to visit and practice holding babies.

"Fat? Fat," she repeated, confused. We said it a number of times. Finally, her eyes brightened. "Oh, *făa fàet*," she said, which sounded identical to our atonal ears. "In Thai, *făa fàet* means twins," she said giggling.

Chris sighed. "I'm such an idiot. Looks like I won't be walking by that corner anytime soon."

"*Mai pen rai*," she said. "Thais don't stay angry."

HOW LONG WERE THOSE DRUNKEN WOMEN HOLDING OUR BABIES?

I know you're not supposed to compare your children. But when you have twins, that's the equivalent of watching the

Olympic finals of the 100-meters and saying, "All the racers looked good to me, even the guy who fell two steps into the sprint. I don't care who broke the world record." I'm not going to go all Tiger Mom here and suggest we put our children on podiums and rank them according to their performances. I prefer Tigger Mom: the energetic, encouraging kind who can pounce if need be and then run far away.

Still, when your girl twin has been smiling for three weeks and your boy twin still doesn't so much as smirk, you start to study the starting blocks.

William, of course, eventually smiled. Actually, he didn't so much smile as grin, showcasing one gorgeous dimple on his left cheek. The problem, however, was that he smiled for *things*: ceiling fans, chrome accessories such as chair legs, and wild patterns. But me? Nothing. I performed "Itsy Bitsy Spider" as a melodrama, I played peek-a-boo as though I were the understudy of a face contortionist, I sneezed like Donald Duck.

Nothing.

I said to Chris, "If I tape tin foil to my face, do you think he'll smile at me?"

"Not likely," he said. "But I would."

"That's not the trophy I'm after, you know."

Then something happened in the shower.

Not conception.

Not William's smile.

Not me seeing my feet after months of having a belly that had me questioning their existence.

But the exfoliation of my stretch marks. It wasn't pretty. They were bright red and wrinkled after the birth. Then one day, I managed a shower when Chris was home. This meant that I didn't have two babies in bouncy chairs on the bathroom floor, squawking a never-ending chorus. I had time to use the best shower weapon there is, the loofah, that naughty sponge.

I scrubbed. And the red, wrinkly stretch marks came off. In their place were these silvery-white stretch marks that glow in the dark, like the reflectors framing a dead-end sign on an abandoned country road.

I kept scrubbing. More kept coming off. It was exhilarating and disgusting, like picking a scab or—worse—watching a teen pregnancy reality show while picking a scab.

I hated those saggy red marks. "Battle scars," Chris called them affectionately. Years later, when Vivian was three, she rechristened them "silver rainbows."

Yet that morning I scoured. And hoped they'd disappear.

I got out of the shower and dressed, making it an auspicious day.

"My stretch marks are shedding," I told Chris.

"Really?"

"Yup, it's Exfoliation Station in the shower. Enter at your own risk."

"I think I'll stay out."

"Good choice. You know," I added, "I'm pretty sure teen moms don't have problems with stretch marks."

"Maybe. But they have a lot of other problems."

"Yes," I said, plugging a pacifier into a fussy twin's mouth, "they do." I entered a reverie wondering how I could have coped with all this fifteen years earlier when I was a teen. I was barely coping as a thirty-three-year-old in a stable marriage. There were women stronger than me, that fact I knew.

I also knew I was glad I didn't have to be stronger than I already was.

Vivian was born an extrovert. When she was still in the hospital nursery, I would always find her because she could out-scream the other four-dozen criers. She liked to speak loudly, even then.

"Like her mother," Chris said.

Vivian and William were the only two wrinkly things in the nursery without a shock of hair. Thai babies are adorable, tending to be born with this gorgeous black hair that almost seems to have been backcombed with salon-quality products. Our kids had wisps of hair in a bad Donald Trump-like comb over.

"Like their mother," Chris teased.

I would've argued had he been wrong, but pregnancy and Franck had taught me I had hair issues.

After we got our spawn home, their hair grew in bizarre patterns, changing each month. Vivian was a Baby Gaga, ahead of her time. At first, her new growth covered her temples and forehead in fine patches.

"When she's older," I told Chris, "she can get her forehead waxed."

Later, that hair fell out and in grew a blond, Krusty the Klown fringe. Later still, she shed that, and new hair grew in the opposite pattern: a military flat top. Finally, near her first birthday, Vivian's hair follicles had a meeting and decided on a coordinated release date.

William's issues were of the neck variety. When we weren't referring to him as "the guy," we called him Torticollis Boy.

Torticollis, or wryneck, is a condition some babies are born with when their neck muscles are stiff or undeveloped on one side, making them twist their head more to the other. Sometimes, it's caused by lack of movement in utero, like in William's case, because his sister spent numerous months practicing her Thai kickboxing, wedging her bigger brother into a tiny corner of the womb. It's no wonder Will was born first; I would've headed out as soon as possible too.

For the first few months, we swaddled Torticollis Boy for his nap; this would stop him from whacking himself or his sister. With his arms and legs wrapped securely and his head tilted to the side and far back, he had quite a unique silhouette.

"He looks like a human Pez dispenser," I said to Chris.

We both doubled over laughing.

Because he did.

We decided to take our Pez dispenser and his sister on an outing to the Thai countryside. Attempting to do a day trip from Bangkok was ambitious since it sometimes took half a day to leave the city. We hired a car and a driver, and headed out to some areas that made and sold pottery.

After two hours of passing by street vendors selling lottery tickets and T-shirts, hearing two-stroke motorcycles roar past us, and looking at foreign men drinking morning beer with young Thai girls, we arrived in the countryside.

I shifted my hips, neatly crammed between Vivian and William's rear-facing car seats, while Chris and our driver discussed how corrupt the Thai police force was. William stared silently out the window, observing the world beyond our apartment. Vivian studied the toys suspended from her car seat handle, like an adult preparing for her LSAT.

Parenting Tip: Placing hanging toys over your baby's car seat will help her score 6423 on her SATs.

I was squished and silent in Quiet Land.

Then we arrived at the pottery village. Within moments, we were offered a trip to a gem factory by another driver's "brother." We wheeled our lucky babies around, bought a few pots, and headed to the car. I performed the never-ending routine: fed babies, changed babies, buckled in babies. *Make babies* ceased to be part of the equation months ago.

As we left the village, Vivian launched into her nails-on-chalkboard series of shrieks with the endurance of a marathon runner. Our driver navigated around an accident—likely caused by a screaming child—and he maneuvered around other developing world road obstacles, like a family of five on a motorbike and a 1960s truck filled with jingling propane bottles. William fell asleep. Vivian kept screaming. Her eyes glanced from me to the window to the other window to her hanging toys to me, never breaking her scream. The moment I shoved a pacifier in her mouth, she spat it out, making it clear that she was no Maggie Simpson.

The tropical rain started, but did little to silence the shrieks. Desperate, I took Vivian's blanket and draped it over her car seat. She stopped crying and we were blessed with silence. I peeked. She was awake but silent.

"What did you do?" Chris asked.

"I put a blanket over the whole car seat."

"Do you think she can still breathe?"

"I hope so."

I peeked again. Child was breathing. Always a good sign.

"It's like she's a bird in a cage and was overstimulated," I said. "Do you think the Birdie Treatment is in any parenting books?"

"I think placing a blanket over my head is an answer to Thailand's chaos," Chris said. Our driver laughed as he slalomed around people packing up their roadside food stalls.

 Parenting Tip: If unable to stop your child from screaming, try the Birdie Treatment. If placing a blanket on the head of your baby doesn't work, try it on yourself.

I laughed too, a forced laugh. I sat in silence and thought about Vivian and her blanket. Maybe that was what I was doing every day: walking around our apartment, around Bangkok, with a blanket over my head every day, not knowing where I was going, not caring if I could see.

Because of the superficial success of Operation Escape Bangkok and a two-week visit from Chris's parents, we left the chaos once again, this time for a weekend. Inside our ubiquitous white tourist van were a driver, my in-laws, Chris, and our five-month-old twins.

It was Vivian and William's longest car journey; from our apartment in Bangkok it was a four-hour drive south to a semiprivate beach near Prachuap Khiri Khan on the Gulf of Thailand. Besides big trucks barreling past us, pedestrians on the side of the highway, and the occasional gathering of police officers, the drive was uneventful. I even managed to stare outside the window for a few miles.

Then we turned off the main highway and headed east on a bumpy road. William and Vivian awoke and started to scream. It was their feeding time, but I told the driver, whose eyes loomed large in the rearview mirror, to keep going. In thirty short minutes, we'd be at the quiet beachside resort.

It was an eternity that no Birdie Treatment could subdue.

I became Animated Mommy, digging into my reserves, anxious to show my loving in-laws that I was a perfect mom. I performed puppet shows, exaggerated facial expressions, and engaged in another Oscar-winning performance of Peek-a-Boo. Finally, I resorted to singing. This is one of those areas I'm less than skilled at. I sang through "Itsy Bitsy Spider," "Mary Had a Little Lamb," and four verses of "Amazing Grace" to the theme song from *Gilligan's Island.*

Chris and his parents joined the choir when I started "Five Little Monkeys Jumping on the Bed." We were at "three little monkeys" when our van pulled out to pass a motorcycle. I looked out the window, looked again to refocus, and stopped singing. I believe I sang something like "one fell off and—what the hell?"

A monkey, a real *live* monkey, was riding on the back of the motorcycle, his little paws on the waist of the driver. Or at least that was what I thought I'd seen. Maybe I'd been inhaling too much exhaust. For a moment, we were suspended in silence. The singing had stopped.

"Was that a monkey driving a motorcycle?" I asked.

Someone nodded. And then my two little monkeys started screaming.

At those beach huts in Prachuap Khiri Khan, I relaxed. Our three-roomed air-conditioned hut was right on the Gulf of

Thailand. I'd sit on the shaded porch while William and Vivian napped inside, and I'd think. Not about abandoning my children, but about nothing. Maybe I could do this parenting thing. Heck, I *was* doing this parenting thing.

After a quick swim where I played avoid-the-jellyfish, I needed to shower and change. Chris entertained our babes on the porch, juggling various squeaky toys to the delights of his audience. I went in. It seemed safe enough.

Ten minutes later, I emerged and saw three women swaying and cooing at our babies. Only William and Vivian weren't on the blanket, but in the arms of two of the women. They were having the time of their lives and, judging from our twins' smiles, so were they. I noticed their friend was holding three Singha beers.

I did what any responsible and concerned mother would do: I grabbed my camera and commemorated the drunken women holding my children.

They kissed our babies, placed them into our arms, and took a swig of their beers. All three friends wandered away, waving and blowing kisses.

"How long were those drunken women holding our babies?" I asked.

"I don't know," said Chris. "About five or ten minutes, I'd say. They were really nice."

WE TRAVEL WITH OUR OWN DUAL AIRBAGS

Back in Bangkok, we put Chris's parents on a plane and returned to our lives, which became routine. Fall—even though no such season existed in Southeast Asia—marched on. Soon, Thanksgiving arrived. We were celebrating it with American friends by cranking up the air conditioner and cooking a turkey.

Well, *we* weren't cooking a turkey; we hadn't even used our oven once in four years and weren't sure if it worked, let alone if it fit a dead bird that wasn't a pigeon who crapped on our balcony. We were getting our twins ready for the party. I was cutting Vivian's nails, body parts which seemed eerily similar to her skin. She already had mutilated herself with numerous scratch marks, so I knew this clipping was overdue.

I sat her wriggly bottom on my lap, put one of her pudgy hands on the table, and began to clip. The first four finger-nails were successful. Then I shifted her hand to clip her thumbnail. Pudgy skin was everywhere. I lined up the nail clippers and, like a batter eying a pitcher, determined my target. Then I swung. Rather blindly.

"#$%*, I cut off her thumb," I screamed. Vivian screamed. We all screamed-together-screamed.

"#$%*, get me some Kleenex. She's bleeding out." Exaggeration is my specialty in a moment of crisis.

Chris deposited William in a bouncy chair and brought me a large box of tissues.

Vivian, of course, had discovered that warrior part of her-self and was screaming bloody murder, which it nearly was.

Chris inspected it.

"You just cut the top off," he said, "that's all."

"That's all?" I said through tears. "I can't do this anymore."

I put Vivian in his arms, collapsed in the chair, and put my head on the table and cried.

"Can't do what?" he asked. "Be a mom?"

I looked up. "I don't know."

"What don't you know?" Chris was now standing, bouncing Vivian around and using even more tissues to stop her from bleeding out.

"I don't know what I don't know."

"Can you offer me any more information?" Chris asked, still bouncing Vivian, who was starting to swallow her sobs and her snot.

I sat up and wiped my eyes. "I know I can't cut their nails anymore. That's the only thing I know for sure."

"No problem," Chris said. "I'll do it."

"And William's?"

"Yes, his too."

"Here." I gave him the clippers. "Her left hand still needs to be done."

"Got it," he said. "I'll try my best to leave her thumb intact."

I forced a smile.

 Parenting Tip: If you maim your child, your spouse will help you out more.

I got through Thanksgiving with a weight on my chest, a weight that made me wonder who I was. I was supposed to be a happy mother, but I was a lump who breastfed her babies and then watched them play, day after endless day. I supposedly led a charmed life. I lived in one of Asia's most exciting cities, and I had a maid who did laundry and cooked for us every weekday. All I had to do was look after two healthy babies.

Only they didn't need much looking after. They didn't even crawl yet. They weren't getting into trouble. I just sat in the living room under the ceiling fans watching them and wondering, *Is this it?*

I rallied a bit in December. We'd decided to go home to Canada for a few weeks. In retrospect, it was an auspicious decision, given that our Plan B option was to fly to Southern Thailand and stay in a hotel that would be ravaged by the Boxing Day tsunami. Without the ability to see into the future, our petty, pre-Christmas concerns dominated our lives as we prepared to fly home to Canada for the holidays.

It was good to have something to do other than stare at cute babies day after day. My sense of humor even returned. I had started going to the Bangkok Twins-and-Triplets playgroup. Other moms with older multiples assured me that the first four months of raising twins were horrible, the next two months were difficult, but after six months it all became *fun*. Like the experts who predicted the housing bubble wouldn't burst, they were wrong. A multi-day flight for four people in two seats was not fun.

Neither was packing, which became the one task I had to focus on. How do you pack for a 120-degree drop in temperature? I tried to recall that algebra class I took a generation ago in order to determine just how many diapers are needed by two babies going on three flights that span thirty hours. I couldn't even find X, let alone solve for it.

I went to find Chris, who was in our bedroom packing for himself.

"Are twenty-eight diapers enough for three flights that take over twenty-four hours?"

"Twenty-eight?" he repeated, pausing from folding his underwear into perfect squares. "For both kids?"

"Yes, for both kids. I'm not planning to bring fifty-eight diapers."

"Fifty-six," he said.

"What?"

"Fifty-six is the double of twenty-eight."

"Never mind. I'll figure it out myself. Do you think I should pack *What To Expect in the First Year*?" I asked. That book rarely left my side.

"I think we can do without it for three weeks," Chris said. "Do you?"

"Umm, I guess so. It's pretty heavy."

"Look," Chris offered, sensing my worry. "If we really need one, we'll buy another at home."

For a few nights prior to the departure of our transpacific flight, I had nightmares of passengers pushing my family out the emergency door, without parachutes. This was what I was thinking when a taxi dropped us off at the Don Muang International Airport amid the chaos of Bangkok.

Being parents, we boarded early so we could keep our babies cooped up in an enclosed space even longer. As we sat on the tarmac, we watched innocent passengers struggle down the aisle to our row, recheck their boarding passes in disbelief, and wonder what they did to get such bad karma.

"They're twins?" they uttered incredulously. "Have they flown before?"

"Nope," I answered.

"Guess you lost the seat lottery," Chris added in a preemptive attempt to build good will. "Bet you're sorry you requested the bulkhead now."

Nervous laughter lessened the tension for a nanosecond, until Vivian tested the speed of sound. With eyes the size of SpongeBob's, she let out a scream that had even me looking around, desperately pretending she wasn't my kid.

William remained unfazed by his sister's screams and opted to employ a more underhanded method of annoyance. He started a dramatic monologue that consisted of yelling the syllable "da" relentlessly at varying pitches. It was cute for the first four seconds.

A flight attendant approached us and demonstrated how to hold our babies for takeoff and landing.

"I think we got it," I said, interrupting her.

She didn't look impressed.

All this occurred before the plane even left the tarmac.

But depart it did. The other 546 passengers became aware of the elevation change meter by meter, thanks to our babies. For the adults, Vivian and William's screams reached high annoyance levels, in the same league as having the Minipops' version of the song "Let's Get It Started" looping in your head. I managed to balance a twin and wrench my wrist to check my watch: one hour had passed since we boarded the cattle car.

Somehow time inched forward. We negotiated several diaper changes in cupboard-sized bathrooms, all of which were as easy as doing a gymnastics routine in a closed coffin.

There is nothing like straddling a toilet, pinning a squirmy kid onto a cafeteria-tray table, and searching for diaper cream at the bottom of a backpack that is floating in urine on the floor. Then repeat with the second kid. How I escaped the cubicle without flushing a child down the toilet, I'll never know. I'm pretty sure the Earth's population would be over eight billion by now if numerous babies hadn't accidentally been flushed down airplane toilets.

Parenting Tip: If you need assistance while changing a baby's diaper in an airplane bathroom, light a cigarette.

Later, after three more hours of crying and a couple of episodes involving passengers and vomit, there was silence. Vivian and William had fallen asleep in their adjacent Cabbage Patch–sized bassinets, hanging from the wall like tents secured to Everest's rock face. A quick glance at the video monitor revealed that we'd crossed the date line. Yes, that infamous Saturday stretched on, like Britney Spears's career. A dozen diaper changes later and two more hours of screaming, we descended.

As the plane skidded to a halt, we managed to keep William and Vivian's heads from smashing into the wall in front of us. The seatbelt sign dinged, we gathered our gear, and trudged up the aisle, whacking "passengers in need of assistance" with bags. If they didn't need help before, they needed it now.

I could wax poetic about how our Dynamic Duo, whose body weight compared with that of an average holiday turkey, were a lesson in adaptability and resilience. But the truth was becoming clear: These two pieces of extra baggage were better travelers than their parents.

Getting off the plane in Winnipeg, one of the coldest cities in the world, was not a breath of fresh air, unless the air you were breathing was liquid nitrogen.

We took our baggage, including the nonhuman variety, and struggled to the luggage carousels where we were met by my extended family carrying snowsuits, car seats, and all other winter gear with the exception of portable igloos.

We handed our spawn over for cuddles, and then we spent an hour stuffing William and Vivian and their limbs inside snow gear, trying not to zip up their chins.

We repeated this charade multiple times over the next two weeks.

In fact, of the three weeks we were in Canada, we spent one week sleeping, one week talking, and one week putting babies in and out of snowsuits.

On our last Sunday at home, Chris and his mom left the house ahead of me, carrying our winterized children. I came out and saw Vivian and William lying on their backs, staring at the sky.

"You can't just throw them in a snow bank," I said to Chris.

"It's for a purpose," he said.

I watched as his mom took a picture.

"See?" Chris added. "They're snow angels."

I smiled. It was good to be home.

Parenting Tip: To entertain passersby or family members, place your baby in a snow bank. Then hide.

But good didn't last long enough. It was time to go back to Asia.

I packed and repacked diapers.

"It'll never happen," Chris said to me, continuing a conversation we'd started earlier.

His parents were entertaining William and Vivian—no doubt stopping them from pulling the tinsel off the Christmas tree—while we struggled to pack our hockey duffels, also known as Canadian suitcases.

"I'm going to call the airline," I said.

"Go wild," Chris said. "But they're not going to upgrade us. Like I said, it'll never happen."

I took his adult double-dog-dare-you, and I called from the other room.

I pranced back into our bedroom. "Can you believe it? They upgraded us to business class. Do you think they meant the babies too?"

"You really think they'll make us leave them in economy?"

"I don't know," I said.

"Did you ask the person you talked to?"

"Not directly. The kids are listed on our tickets and their seats are on our laps, so I'm pretty sure it's OK," I said. "Anyway, since the vouchers are good for just one flight, we're only upgraded for the Vancouver–Hong Kong leg."

"Isn't that the thirteen-hour flight?"

"Yes."

"Well, that's the one that matters."

One day later, we transferred from our domestic flight in Vancouver and joined business class with our babies.

All the suits gasped.

"They're twins," I volunteered. "We travel with our own dual airbags."

I fake smiled.

And fake prayed.

Then the announcement came, the one that was worse than *prepare for a crash landing*.

"This is your First Officer Tyler. We are currently in line to have the plane de-iced. We estimate we will be delayed ninety minutes. Our crew will be around to offer you drink service."

I pulled out a boob. I was the drink service for my kids.

Once everyone was drunk, the mood softened.

Under the threat of sleeping in the overhead bin, Vivian and William behaved and slept. When they weren't sleeping, drunk people in suits held them.

As long as they were content, I didn't care.

I'M SCREWING UP OUR KIDS

Not long after returning to Thailand and adjusting to the twelve-hour time difference, it hit me full force: Postpartum Depression. Only I didn't know it was PPD, because my twins were seven months old.

I couldn't sleep. At all.

Or eat.

Or think.
Or find anything funny.

Google and a friend helped diagnose me.
More people helped me get better, including doctors and counselors.

It took longer than this page.
It took months.

I have very few memories of that time, except one enduring fear that I told Chris. "I'm screwing up our kids."
"No you're not," he said.

He was right. It took months—and a team of people—for me to believe that.
When I emerged out of my dark cocoon, I tossed the rest of the parenting books out.

Parenting Tip: Everything is a stage. It will pass. Just like that penny your baby ingested.

WE'RE SCARRING THEM FOR LIFE

When Vivian and William were closing in on turning one and I had rediscovered some of my ability to laugh, we decided to go on one final family vacation in Thailand, mostly because we didn't know any better. We boarded a plane in Bangkok and survived a one-hour flight to Chiang Mai, a laid back city in northern Thailand.

The week went well enough, if you consider the following facts:

- We rarely left the dusty room of our guesthouse.
- We were in bed by 6:30 each night, because that's when our twins conked out.
- We had five toys with us and had to entertain two kids with them.
- Guesthouses are not baby proof; they're not even adult proof. They're outfitted with lamp cords, electrical sockets and dangling wires, and bizarre hot water heaters that would send a certified electrician into cardiac arrest.
- A ten-month-old baby is mobile; ten-month-old twins are a roaming gang. One moment they're there, the next they're gone. It's a magic show brought to you by Pampers.

I kind of coped. Maybe it was because I got a lot of sleep, something that had been rare in the past three months.

Everything went well enough, at least until we arrived at the Chiang Mai Airport.

After checking our luggage, car seats, booster seats, and three suitcases of soiled laundry, we wheeled our stroller to the gate. We collapsed into two chairs and freed William and Vivian from captivity. They crawled around the carpeted floor, weaving in and out of a multi-leg obstacle course.

Soon, I was chatting with people nearby, answering questions about twins, claiming that our first vacation had been a success.

Chris was talking to a California tourist who owned a weight loss clinic. The doctor was the color orange.

Eventually I remembered I had children. I spotted Vivian. Then I looked for William.

"God help me," I said. "He's sucking on the stroller wheel."

Yes, the year after the SARS outbreak, our twins were not only crawling around a carpeted airport floor in a developing country, but one twin was sucking on the same stroller that, the day before, had been bumping its way over basketball-sized dung at the elephant orphanage.

The other passengers-in-waiting looked in horror at William lip-locked with the stroller wheel. I stumbled over, broke the suction, and picked him up.

I picked up a pacifier I found in the bottom of the diaper bag and plopped it in his mouth. And thus ended the days of sterilizing anything. Even my wine glass.

 Parenting Tip: When your baby starts sucking on the stroller wheel, it's acceptable to stop sterilizing and to start drinking.

Only weeks after returning to our Bangkok apartment, it was time to start packing. For good this time.

Vivian and William had learned to walk, kind of. They'd each grab the handle of a plastic toy shopping cart for balance, and they'd roam around our large apartment and have their own demolition derby. In retrospect, we should've put helmets on them: A thin layer of parquet flooring does little to soften the concrete beneath. Once again, though, William and Vivian survived.

Packing up eight years of living overseas sucked. To pack the breakables, we hired professional movers—an oxymoron meaning people who place one thing inside each box so they can charge more. Chris, however, opted to pack our summer clothes that would never again be worn. He also packed his books and DVDs. Because nothing makes more sense than shipping a thousand books and DVDs overseas.

Chris started Operation Box Construction, which involved packing tape and a utility knife, two items that can get eleven-month-old twins into a lot of trouble. I did what a loving wife would do: I sent him to another room.

But it wasn't the knife that would destroy Vivian and William. It was the sound of packing tape being unleashed from the roll. If the act of tearing off a Band-Aid made a sound, it would be that of packing tape. As soon as Chris unleashed an arm's length of tape, William and Vivian would go into high pitched, incessant screams, as though they were being mauled by a cat, an angry cat that was having its hair knit into a blanket.

Chris, being in the other room, ignored the screams. He hadn't quite figured out the cause and effect. So, with one twin on each hip, I kicked open the door.

"Stop," I said.

"Stop what?" he said, looking up at our two sobbing spawn who were using my tank top as a tissue.

"The tape. We're scarring them for life. Even more than we already have."

"Really?" he said. "You mean this?" And he launched another three feet of tape. Hysterics followed. Some belonged to Vivian and William.

"You're going to have to move onto the balcony," I said when I'd calmed down.

"Really?"

"Yes."

Chris smiled. "Do you mean to make boxes or to sleep?"

"That depends," I said. "Have you packed the hammock?"

THE SAPPY FILES, PART 2 (OR WHY MY KIDS' FUTURE THERAPISTS SHOULD BELIEVE I'M SOMEWHAT SANE)

Dear William and Vivian,

Happy first birthday. You two seem to have thrived during this year, in spite of our made-up parenting style and the fact that I don't remember much of the second half of your first year.

Do you know that we didn't even throw a first birthday party for you? It didn't seem to make sense to go to all that trouble given that our shipment had gone back to Canada, we had ten days left in Thailand, and you weren't exactly going to remember a party.

My lovely friend Sarah, however, invited us across the hall for birthday celebrations. Yes, she had made you a cake. She's part of the village that is raising you.

Her kindness reminds me of our friend Kaye, a funky and kind Australian grandma-type. When you were only a few weeks old, Kaye visited and cradled one of you, and she told us this: "When they're this little, you just give and give and give. You give so much you don't think you have anything left to give. And you get nothing in return." She wiggled your toes. "But then, starting around six weeks old, you start getting something. A smile, perhaps. Recognition. And from that point on, you start getting back. And you know what? You just keep getting from them. They give you so much in return."

I think I sighed loudly.

"Hang on," Kaye told me. "You'll get there. And then you will keep getting."

I've always remembered that. And you know what? She's right. Your dad and I have started getting. I was even getting when I was in my fog, my depression. Do you know that during my many insomniac nights I would sneak into your room and lie on the floor? You both gave me the gift of a moment's peace. Your deep breaths somehow told me that things were going to be OK. And now, from your giggles to your pick-me-up stance, we are getting so much. Maybe not more than we're giving. Let's face it; there are days when I still want to throw myself in front of a tuk tuk. But I'm getting things back. And I'm going to stop keeping score. Promise. Kind of.

Welcome to One.

I love you both.

Mommy

PART THREE

THE TODDLER YEARS, OR REASONS TO START A THERAPY FUND

CHAPTER 7

THE TODDLER YEARS, OR REASONS TO START A THERAPY FUND

WE NEED TO OUTWIT, OUTLAST, OUTNUMBER OUR KIDS

If we thought flying with our dual airbags the first time was difficult, we were wrong. Now that William and Vivian were doing the drunken baby walk, this transpacific flight was like summiting Everest without the assistance of oxygen, *sherpas*, or our nanny.

Still, some things went our way. Although the check-in agent wouldn't let our one-year-old twins fly in dog crates, she compensated by ignoring the weight of our hockey duffels and let the four of us wave bye-bye to our luggage. Vivian and William's permanent passports had arrived before we left and even though they looked like one-year-old criminal masterminds, security let them through.

After a flight attendant listened to my life story, she doubled our seat allowance by giving us four seats in the middle row, with Chris and I serving as bookends to our babies near the bowels of the aircraft. We each had to hold a baby for takeoff. I believe airlines are conducting an ongoing study about the strength of parents' arms in the event of a crash. I suspect physics wins, every time.

Chris looked at me and joked, "Should we try to stuff them into the overhead bins?"

I laughed. "Maybe. But do you want to play Catch-the-Baby at 38,000 feet?"

Once all our eardrums were blown from air pressure, three of us dozed. I still wasn't great at this sleep thing, but I could help achieve it in others. I broke every airline code and parenting oath by placing William and Vivian on the floor. I plunked them down at our feet, shoved pacifiers into their mouths, and put the tray tables down to hide our babies from flight attendants. I figured under the seat in front of me was safer than the overhead bins. Then, with two live foot warmers asleep on my toes, I relaxed by comparing pictures of Colin Firth in gossip magazines.

There were worse ways of passing time while flying. One was when your children awoke. Vivian and William were truly toddlers at this point, wanting to move when awake. So they waddled up and down the aisles doing the baby shuffle. I'm pretty sure airplane armrests were designed to give barely mobile kids as many black eyes as possible.

They walked. They fell. They entertained other passengers, who smiled either because our babies were adorable in their topsy-turvy way or because the airplane meal-of-the-moment gave everyone gas they were trying to expel.

Eventually more food and drink carts charged down the aisle, corralling William and Vivian. Our kids were now moments away from realizing that those silver airplane zambonis contained the keys to the kingdom: processed food.

A flight attendant rammed her cart into my leg. She said something like, "Would you prefer the dried-out cookies or the carcinogenic pretzel-crap?"

I ordered the peanuts. She winced. "We don't have pea-nuts anymore due to allergies."

Right. "I'll have the cookies," I mumbled.

"And your children?" she asked.

I looked at Vivian and William. Vivian was tearing apart the in-flight magazine and William was flinging every book and toy we'd brought around the cabin. I paused. Our kids had never eaten anything processed. Even though I'd thrown out the parenting books, I still hadn't completely let go of the idea of perfection parenting. The only dessert our twins had ever eaten was a teaspoon of chocolate birthday cake two weeks before and even that had been homemade.

William started pounding on the seat in front of him. I looked at Chris and raised my eyebrows, which are capa-ble of holding entire conversations on their own. Chris shrugged in return, a movement I interpreted as "Why not?"

I took the prepackaged cookies, opened them, and watched as William, Vivian, and their salivary glands dis-covered cookie nirvana. An hour later, I went back to the zamboni cart for more.

 Parenting Tip: On long trips, let your children eat whatever processed crap you can get your hands on.

The final leg of our thirty-hour homeward journey just about killed me. I no longer cared what Vivian and William were up to. I reverted to my not-coping strategy of hum-ming "Jesus Loves Me," this time while banging the seat in front of me. It was a mini-asylum at 38,000 feet for a Sunday school alumnus. Hello, Postpartum Aggression.

We landed in summery Winnipeg, home of the world's biggest mosquitoes, an NHL team that had grown tired of winter and relocated to Phoenix, and my family.

We had two weeks to visit and recover from a twelve-hour time difference before we moved in with Chris's parents in Alberta—800 miles west of Manitoba—where we'd live until I found a teaching job.

Miraculously, while still in Manitoba, I had a telephone interview for a fantastic teaching gig near Calgary. Not so miraculously, I didn't get it. It was for a Drama/English position, and it wasn't hard to figure out that I didn't have much experience in theater. Apparently, raising twins while suffering from Postpartum Depression does not count as *drama*.

Finally, we arrived at my in-laws', where we moved in. We were pseudo-homeless, rather jobless, and no one could sleep through the night. In spite of this, we were welcomed, even if my father-in-law counted the days we stayed there and announced the tally every evening as a joke.

"It's Day Thirteen," he said, handing me a beer.

I chuckled, opened the can, and toasted the baker's dozen of days we'd been there. My husband's father never had beer in the fridge, but he always bought some for me when I visited. We'd sit there, drink a can, and spend a lot of time laughing. I knew he loved me as a daughter.

Chris and his mom joined us in the living room, watching William and Vivian put 1960s era toys coated with lead-based paint in their mouths. But hey, they'd sucked stroller wheels and survived.

"There's going to be a lot of screaming tonight," I announced.

Everyone stopped and looked at me. Even our twins froze, like they could sense something foreboding.

"I apologize in advance," I said, pausing to take a swig of beer. "But I need them to sleep through the night." I pointed to Vivian and William with my foot.

People nodded slowly, computing what this meant for them.

"We're crying it out," I said with the finality of a jail cell closing.

Crying it out was precisely what the kids and I did. Ninety minutes of one twin or the other screaming from 2 AM on. Every two minutes I'd walk into their room, lay them down, and pat their bums for a minute. Then I'd leave. I'd add a minute each time, letting them cry longer. I had nerves of steel, for the first twelve minutes. Chris joined me on the steps, and we chatted while our babies cried.

"Remember the show *Survivor*?" I asked.

Chris nodded.

"That's what parenting is like," I said. "We need to outwit, outlast, outnumber our kids. That's what we're doing now."

"I don't think *outnumber* is part of *Survivor*'s motto. If it is, we should've only had one kid," Chris said.

I shrugged. "If we stopped at one kid, there'd still be one in my uterus."

Parenting Tip: To help you survive raising children, you need to "outwit, outplay, outlast" them each day. Or hire a babysitter.

I looked at my watch. Fifteen minutes had passed. "Time to go pat some bums," I said. We walked into the room together and each patted a little bum, reminding our babes we hadn't abandoned them forever. At 3:30 AM they fell asleep. At 3:31 AM we fell asleep too.

"Do you think your parents hate me?" I said to Chris the next morning while we each dressed a kid.

"Hate? No, they could never hate you. They're probably very tired though. And dreaming about a quiet hotel room."

"I dream about a quiet hotel room too," I said.

"Is that so?" Chris asked suggestively.

"For sleeping," I clarified. "By myself."

I sighed, walked to the kitchen with a kid on each hip, and deposited Vivian and William with their grandparents.

"Night Thirteen was a long one, wasn't it?" I said, plugging in the kettle.

"Just a little noisy," Chris's mom said.

"Well," I said, "you may wish to nap because we're doing it again."

Night Fourteen yielded twenty minutes of crying and bum-patting.

Night Fifteen resulted in two minutes of crying.

And from Night Sixteen on, both twins slept through the night. And so did their mom.

On Day Seventeen, I had a job interview in Calgary, Canada's oil and gas hub. If my in-laws thought that the previous nights had been long, their day just got longer. They had the twins for nine hours while we drove 180 miles to the interview and back. At 8 AM on Day Eighteen, the phone rang. It was for me. I took a sip of tea, handed off a kid, and took the receiver from my mother-in-law. I had landed a great teaching job.

Chris and I spent three days looking at thirty-six houses with a real estate agent who doubled as a babysitter before we found a home I liked. We got possession of our suburban abode after spending Day Forty-Eight with my in-laws.

"If you count part days, it was technically forty-nine," my father-in-law joked.

"It didn't feel less than eighty-two," I said, giving him a goodbye hug.

I'M SWEARING MY WAY TO CLEANLINESS

We moved into our new house without furniture. Nothing makes a first night in a city where you know no one more welcoming than two sleeping bags on the floor of a curtainless master bedroom when the sun doesn't set until 10 PM.

Chris bought us a bed the next day.

Vivian and William fared better. When we moved back to Canada, we didn't bother shipping their two cribs. First, we didn't know if they would meet Canadian standards, and we didn't want the Royal Canadian Mounted Police to ride up on their steeds, inspect the width between the crib bars, and haul the beds away. Instead, we shipped two playpens that didn't meet North American standards either. At least our little suckers had beds.

Settling in was difficult. I spent the first week crawling after William and Vivian, shoving plug protectors into electrical outlets before our babies channeled their inner Benjamin Franklin. Chris, meanwhile, assembled IKEA furniture for the duration it would take a drunk person to say,

"Allen key" six billion times. We also put up mini crowd-control gates everywhere, turning the first floor of our house into a baby Alcatraz.

We went on outings, too, trying to find things in our quiet suburb, like a bank. We were there setting up accounts, getting credit cards, and ensuring our mortgage wasn't going to have us eating at the soup kitchen. It was all a little depressing.

We were loading Vivian and William back into their car seats when I confessed to Chris. "I robbed the bank."

"Yeah, right," he said.

"No, really," I said. "I stole something."

"A pen?"

"Better. Much, much better."

I shut the rear door and climbed into the passenger seat. "It's in here," I said, motioning to the diaper bag.

"Let's see the bounty," Chris said.

I pulled out a phonebook and flashed my best Ma Barker smile.

 Parenting Tip: If you rob a bank, don't brag about it in front of your children or in a book.

We'd been told the previous day that the city was out of phonebooks and that we wouldn't be able to get any until November. Given that neither of us had a smart phone, this proved challenging. How could you call the Internet providers or cable companies if you couldn't find their phone number?

"Well done," Chris said. "It's not quite as big as the flower arrangements you used to walk out of Bangkok hotels with. Remember? You'd even get the security guards to help you."

I nodded. Maybe the next time I'd steal a plant. We didn't have any of those either.

Our first "fun" family outing was to the zoo. It was nearing the end of August. The temperature was 65°F when we arrived. Within two hours, the mercury plummeted to 39°F.

William and Vivian were not only being chased by free-roaming peacocks, they were shivering. Snow clouds gathered in the sky. "What kind of city did you move us to?" I asked Chris.

"One with a mountainous climate."

"We aren't in Bangkok anymore, that's for sure," I said. "I want our nanny. Or at least a winter coat."

The night before I started teaching, I decided to quit breast-feeding. Vivian and William were fifteen months old and pretty unimpressed with this whole boob thing. For the previous week, I'd been waking them up at 10 PM for their only feed of the day. With them drinking cow's milk out of glasses, my udders became redundant.

My timing could have been better. I could have waited for a long weekend or for any weekend. But I didn't. So by the second day of school, I was engorged and desperately praying I didn't see a baby anywhere. I wore three shirts and five breast pads just in case.

One night after putting our kids to bed, I was cleaning the kitchen and about to start on a mountain of grading.

"What's that thumping?" Chris asked.

I paused hockey practice, my euphemism for sweeping. Our house came with a VacPan—an automatic dust pan in the kitchen—which made sweeping a sport. Abandoned Cheerios made great pucks, the broom a decent hockey stick, the VacPan a net. I was perfecting my broom slap shot. The fact that my ratio of crushed Cheerios to actual goals was 3:1 did not deter me.

This day, however, I scored. "She shoots, she scores!"

I noticed Chris looking at me oddly. It could've been because I was celebrating by playing air guitar with the broom. I shut off the VacPan with my toe. "Did you say something?" I asked.

"Listen to the thumping. What is it?"

I heard a series of uneven staccato beats. Our ceiling light shook.

"It's just the kids. They're bunny-hopping their playpens across the room."

"Really?"

"Yup. They started doing it last weekend during naptime. It's quite funny to see."

We snuck upstairs and peeked in their room. Sure enough, William and Vivian were each standing in their playpens, legs wide apart, one hand grasping each side, and bunny-hopping their playpens across the room. It was like a sack race at a church picnic. Once they'd reach the wall, they'd pivot their bodies around and hop back.

William saw us standing at the doorway. Our sleeper-clad hopper paused and then burst into giggles. Vivian followed.

I shook my head. "No more racing tonight," I said. "It's sleep time."

One hour later, they listened. The thumping that remained in my head was caused by reading eighth grade essays.

At various points that autumn, I walked into Vivian and William's room to find unwelcome discoveries. There was the time I found one child sleeping naked beside a massive log of poo. There was the time I found every article of clothing in a heap on the floor, an indoor pile of leaves to jump in. I'd come into their room to find them sleeping in the same playpen. I'd seen carefully constructed postmodernist sculptures, sometimes on each other's heads.

Apparently one sleeping twin was too much for the other to resist. One Saturday, when Vivian should have been napping, she took all forty of the board books in her room and dumped them over sleeping William.

"Did you do this?" I asked Vivian, motioning to the collection of Dr. Seuss and Sandra Boynton on William's face.

Vivian nodded. At least she hadn't inherited my ability to lie convincingly.

"You know," I said, "burying your brother in books is not a good idea."

She giggled. William woke up and emerged from the alphabet rubble. Like a good twin brother, he didn't care; he smiled at the library in his bed and started to paw his way through *Green Eggs and Ham.*

Oh I do not like big messes, gosh damn. I do not like them, Mom I am.

Not long after the playpen and book incidents, William and Vivian escalated their bedroom delinquency. Vivian swung from the mesh, stuffed-animal cylinder that hung from the ceiling by a plant hook. Channeling her inner monkey, she grabbed on and lifted her feet. Around and around she went until she fell and cracked her head on her dresser. I heard the scream; so did our friends in Thailand. There's still a hole in the ceiling's plaster. Vivian's head fared slightly better.

William rebelled artistically. He took the nightlight out of the socket and used the prongs to scratch paint off the wall. Not long after these two incidents, we supervised their naptimes. Chris, who worked from home, would lie down on a comforter between their playpens and pretend to sleep. If they attempted any shenanigans, he'd reach out his zombie hand and grab the delinquent's ankle before the reign of terror began.

Supervised naptime worked well for the first week. And then I took over the weekend nap patrol and was never so well rested. I'd fall asleep before Vivian and William zonked out. It was bliss until I awoke to two giggly faces above me. I put a moratorium on weekend naps, for all of us.

Soon their shenanigans shifted to bedtime. They started opening the closet and pulling everything out. Nothing stopped them. Tired of shoving it all in and attempting to shut the door before more junk tumbled out, I said to Chris, "We need to put a lock on their closet." What I meant was, "You need to put a lock on their closet."

This was not one of those items that sat on the fridge's to-do list for six months; strangely enough, tasks involving a cordless drill rose to the top. Later that day, Chris wielded his second favorite weapon, went out to the back fence, removed the sliding lock, and placed it at the top of their closet.

This worked for one day, until our twins wrenched on the doors so hard that the lock bent. At which point I waved a white towel and got out *my* second favorite tool: the corkscrew.

Chris had a thing with bodily functions: unless they were his own, he had trouble dealing with them. So in our familial dysfunction, I became the go-to person for all things poo and puke related.

This was not in our vows. I always thought writing your own vows was "making it up"; now I think it's wise. If I were to marry again, I would add this to Chris's vows: "I promise to share cleaning the bathrooms, including crap that's smeared on the toilet, pee that's covering the back wall, and chunky trails of puke from the kids' room to our room. I will also give you at least one foot rub a week."

It's a good thing I'm not single.

I've found poo everywhere in our house. In playpens, in underwear, on carpets, and on the tile floor.

All this I handled by hitting my head on the picture window until it bled.

Well, some of the time. Sometimes, I was less composed, like when I was naked. I had just showered. I grabbed a towel off the rack and saw something above the toilet roll dispenser. I squinted and examined it. Poo. Dried, crusty poo. It looked liked some frat boy had tried to faux finish our wall with it.

Both William and Vivian still wore diapers, but I knew their habits of removing dirty ones.

I cranked open the door and yelled, "Who smeared poo on the wall?"

No one answered, so I did what every calm person does in the face of adversity. I wrapped a towel around me and strode down the stairs leaving a trail of water in my wake. I repeated the question.

Both twins looked up from the scribbling they were doing at the table.

They shook their heads.

"Let's see your hands."

Nothing but wash-off marker, the biggest misnomer since Easy Bake ovens graced toy stores.

Chris watched my tirade. He'd learned when to shut it, a Pavlovian non-response that prevented most major marital discord.

I grabbed a pail and the jumbo bottle of Mr. Clean and dripped my way upstairs.

Thirty minutes later, I heard, "You OK?"

"I'm swearing my way to cleanliness."

It was what I did when anger overtook me: I cleaned loudly and swore silently. Usually Chris was the catalyst for my cleaning forays; in fact, I was beginning to think he intentionally pissed me off so I'd scour the house.

First I swore my vows, then I swore my way to cleanliness.

WOULD YOU PUT YOUR PENIS AWAY?

Winter settled in which meant we spent one extra hour every day putting our kids into snowsuits and another extra hour looking for lost mittens. Some people wondered what they used to do with all their time before they had kids. I wondered what we used to do with all our time before we had kids in a wintry climate and before we decided we didn't need a nanny.

That's right, I thought. *I remember what I did. I went loopy because I had nothing to do except read parenting books and wish I were perfect.*

I closed that head movie and wedged boots onto one twin's feet.

It was 5 PM on a weeknight, pitch black outside, and we were taking Vivian and William to get their eighteen-month vaccinations. Nothing said fun like driving fifteen minutes on icy streets to make your children scream.

We weren't completely stupid, however. We had a plan. Wars had been won and lost on logistics, so we'd gone over tonight's mission in scrupulous detail. William would go first. Experience had taught us that he could handle pain. Experience had also taught us that Vivian could handle pain, providing she screamed for sixty consecutive minutes.

William, our beloved introvert, winced when the nurse injected him with the vaccine concoction. Chris dressed him in his winter gear. We'd kept Vivian half dressed in her snowsuit. We were planning to do a jab-and-run with her. She sat on my lap and I held her in a vise-like grip. One-two-three-jab followed by an endless ear-piercing scream. I shoved her flailing arms into the top of her snowsuit, and we made our way to the car. Operation Destroy-the-Sound-Barrier was successful.

Days after this, I became sick, as in can't-go-to-work sick. We didn't yet have a family physician because it was impossible to find a doctor who was accepting patients in this thriving city that everyone was moving to.

But at 8 AM, we tried. With our real estate agent minding our twins, we set off to find a doctor. We pulled up to an office beside our public library, a place I knew because William and Vivian had slobbered over half their board books. Plus, I'd already paid enough fines to fund the library's expansion.

The medical clinic didn't open until 9 AM, but the lights were on. We went in. I told the receptionist my story, which included too much information, like "twins at home," "new to the city," "no family within two hundred miles." She informed me that walk-in hours didn't start until 4 PM. I nodded while tears welled in my eyes and my body shook from a high fever.

"Sit down for a minute," she said, before I passed out. "I'll be right back."

I collapsed into a chair, and Chris rubbed my back before withdrawing his hand for his own coughing attack. A new country meant new germs.

The receptionist returned with a smile. "There's a doctor in doing paperwork. She'll see you both now. Follow me."

We went in together. At the end of both of our examinations, the doctor looked from Chris to me and back to Chris.

She addressed him. "You are sick," she said. "But your wife is much sicker."

I had won the competition. If I'd possessed any energy, I'd have danced on the examination table.

Before we left, I asked, "Are you taking patients?"

"No," she said, "but my colleague is unofficially taking a couple. Talk to the receptionist. She'll set you up."

We nearly skipped our zombie selves out of there.

Calgary was becoming home, one stumble after another.

Soon, we were both on the mend with meds in our system and a doctor for our entire family. William was doing what he did best: building towers, kicking them over, and laughing. Vivian was doing what she did best: practicing things like climbing stairs, talking, and laughing at her brother's antics everywhere, even in the bathroom.

When William and Vivian were toddlers, they shared a bath. This saved both time and water, but destroyed my remaining shreds of sanity. It didn't take me long to realize that there were many scientific lessons that could be learned by bathing children.

1. Friction, or lack thereof, occurred when you picked up your baby out of the bathwater with shampoo-covered hands.

2. Water temperature warmed when your child urinated in it.

3. Density was demonstrated when your child's poo sank to the bottom of the tub.

4. Molds were what came out of squeaky bath toys and under the fat rolls in your baby's neck.

5. Water displacement occurred when water that started in the tub ended up on the floor.

6. Anatomy revealed that girls had vaginas; boys had penises.

7. Several theories were tested, including Newton's Third Law of Motion, which declared that for every action there was always an equal and opposite reaction. So

when kids drank the bath water, Mommy reacted by yelling, "Don't drink the bath water. It's bum water."

8. Saturation occurred when your child's hands wrinkled because you left them in the bath for fifty-six minutes.

9. Spontaneous combustion was demonstrated by the laughter that ensued when one child farted in the bathwater.

10. Conclusions were offered when you realized your husband should bathe the children more often.

My scientific reasoning didn't stop with bath time. In the imaginary PhD thesis I wrote on Darwin and Freud, I determined that women were more highly evolved than men because their sexual organs could not be hacked off or injured as easily. Chris doubted my empirical data, which was every bit as reliable as the study that showed trail mix made with M&Ms trumped trail mix made with Smarties, nine times out of seven.

With a toddler son in the house, the word *penis* is thrown around with great regularity, kind of like the word *tampon* in a Playtex factory. I don't care if you call a phallus a wee-wee, a little peter, or a scrumpadoodle, but it's alive and well in all family units that have Y-chromosomes (by the way, Y = an X that has had part of it chopped off. See? I rest my case).

Most mothers spend part of their day saying, "Would you put your penis away?" or "Can you please go to your bedroom if you want to inspect the goods?"

I too have said this. Sometimes to William. Sometimes to Chris.

MOMMY WILL SNEEZE LIKE DONALD DUCK
IF YOU PICK UP YOUR TOYS

When I was a kid, I was the most popular kid on the block. Since we lived on a farm, I was also the least popular kid on the block being I was the only kid for two miles. Still, my 1970s toys had clout. My Fisher Price collection was impressive, but what my friends really liked was the fact that I had an anatomically correct boy doll. I had inherited this from my older siblings, who were born in the '60s, that era of free love and penises. This was not a doll in the style of a neutered Ken that most of my friends had; it was a fat plump plastic doll with a penis and scrotum.

As a child, I didn't use the word penis. And I may have thought scrotum was a bad infection. Some days I still think this. Regardless of what I did or didn't call these bawdy parts, this doll was the reason I insisted on teaching my kids the correct names for their body parts.

From an early age, my kids knew *penis*, *vagina*, and even *nose*.

So one evening I was more surprised than Nick Nolte when *People* magazine named him the sexiest man alive. William was sitting on my lap. I had just finished reading *The Cat in the Hat* with a British accent when he looked at me and said, "Mommy. Nipples?"

I blurted, "Pardon?"

"Count," William said. "One, two, free, four, five—"

"Whoa, there," I interrupted. "Just what are you counting?"

He pointed first to my neck, then his finger lingered on my cheek.

"That's not a nipple," I said. "It's a mole."

Later that night, after William and his sister were in bed, I searched eBay for an anatomically correct doll. One with both nipples and moles.

Parenting Tip: Buy an anatomically correct doll. It will help your children learn to differentiate moles from nipples, and armpits from butts.

I know some people claim there is no such thing as a stupid question. They lie. Especially when it involves biology.

Every parent is the recipient of stupid questions, but I'm willing to wager my husband that parents of twins get more stupid questions than a politician who's run out of a strip club wearing half a giraffe costume.

The first time it happened was on the campus of the school I taught at in Bangkok. A parent, a particularly bright British parent, walked up to me and offered his congratulations to me and to Vivian and William, who were asleep in the stroller. Then the parent asked, "Are they identical?"

Before you think this wasn't a stupid question, may I just say that William and Vivian were dressed in pink and blue. Yes, Chris and I believed in stereotyping them from their first days on planet Earth.

"No, they're not identical. He—"

He graciously interrupted me.

"But they look identical."

"Well, they share some genetic material since they both carry my DNA."

"They really look identical," he persisted. "Are you sure they're not?"

I could've handled one stupid question. With his follow up, the brash part of my brain took over.

I nodded. "Well, I'm pretty sure. William has a penis, and Vivian has a vagina."

"Right," he said, mildly embarrassed. "But they do look alike."

Of course, so do Dora and Diego when you've only seen them once.

I've had the same conversation multiple times, so many that it makes me wonder what people were thinking of during the sexual reproduction unit in Biology class.

The hillbilly cousin to the "are they identical" question was, *Are they natural?* The public seemed to have a burning desire to know if twins were conceived by fertility treatments or naturally. As if having sex every day and night for four months trying to get pregnant is *natural*.

I got tired of this question too. Depending on my snark-o-meter reading that day, I gave one of six answers:

1. "Yes, they're natural. They breathe air."
2. "Well, they have opposable thumbs, so that's pretty natural."
3. "No, they're not natural. They keep me up all night and make me want to curl up in a ball in my closet."
4. "Well, we limit their exposure to polymers, but we do allow them to eat processed food, including fried baloney, Spam, and Jell-o."

5. "No, they're not natural. They're clothed, at least in public."
6. "They're as natural as your breasts."

Usually, if I replied with any answer other than the first response, Chris would smile and usher me and our children away.

 Parenting Tip: When people ask you stupid questions about your children, it is your right and responsibility to give them stupid answers.

I was one of those pathetic parents who chose to withhold items from my children because it was easier than dealing with trying to limit that thing. Glitter was number one on my list of contraband. It was prohibited from my house, ahead of handguns and illegal drugs. Number two was finger paint; who needs it when you have ketchup, the wonder condiment? Number three was ice cream, possibly because I'd eaten my lifetime quota while living in Bangkok.

When our friend from Texas visited us in Calgary, we took her to the Rocky Mountains. We rode the gondola up Sulphur Mountain and when we disembarked, it was colder than Winnipeg. So, our Texan friend did what all Texans do when they're cold: she bought ice cream. While my twins had eaten ice cream, they'd never had a cone before. Again, we all knew that as parents we needed to be consistent: if I banned glitter and finger paint due to the mess, then it followed that I must prohibit ice cream cones.

But, like the cookies on the airplane, I acquiesced, hoping the new treat might stop William and Vivian from free falling off the side of the 7,500-foot mountain.

We asked them to choose from two flavors: vanilla or vanilla. They chose the latter.

> Parenting Tip: Always give your child the illusion of choice. For your ease, make the two choices identical.

Vivian started by inspecting her ice cream cone from every possible angle, no doubt assessing whether or not she could recreate this creation in a complex craft session at home. While looking at the pointy end, she got a lesson in gravity as the single scoop of ice cream fell. I half caught it and plopped it onto her cone before her screams started an avalanche.

William tested Newton's laws in another way. He decided to eat the cone from the bottom. This was the same boy who bit a giant hole in the middle of his slice of pizza so it resembled a triangular donut.

This time, understatement won as the parenting technique of the moment. "William," I said, "it's usually best not to bite the bottom of the cone first."

Ice cream dripped on the frozen ground, and I restrained him from lapping it up. My Texan friend smiled, once again convinced of her decision not to have children.

> Parenting Tip: Stating the obvious to your children is a gentle introduction to the art of sarcasm.

For our wedding, my parents gave us a lump sum of money. Since Chris and I married in Canada in the middle of a move from Bahrain to Thailand, we opted for an IOU, cashable when we returned to North America.

We used the money to purchase a dining room table and chairs. My best memories of my own family occurred around the dinner table. We had many large gatherings and a lot of laughs. After his first dinner with us, Chris remarked, "It's like eating with Vikings. There's a lot of food, a lot of wine, and it's very, very loud." The only way you were heard at these dinners was if you yelled over the laughter. It was competitive repartee.

A table, then, was a nostalgic gift. To find one I loved, we interviewed furniture makers and chose a Dutch-Canadian family business that made us a beautiful set that cost more than our children. When the furniture makers told us how to care for our table, the Dutch father asked, "How do you plan to use it?"

I told them for every meal. Then I added, "We have twins. They're toddlers."

"It'll see wear and tear then," one of the brothers said. "But furniture should be used." I sensed him mourning his art.

I suspected they knew it'd be abused. Possibly by twins who colored at the table.

With the golden slab of maple in its virginal state, William and Vivian focused on trying to stay on their coloring pages. They were using wash-off markers. Until they weren't.

"That's not—" I started. "It can't be . . . you didn't . . . Move the paper . . . now."

I saw black marker covering a large section the table. "Tell me that's not permanent marker."

Both kids looked at me, big-eyed faces also full of marker.

"Give me those markers," I snapped.

They ran crying into the living room.

They were my Sharpies. For work. And they'd become one with my table.

I was angry so I cleaned.

I pulled out my arsenal: Mr. Clean, Fantastic, soap, lemon, baking powder, vinegar. I made a volcano with the last two. All of these methods were Helpful Hints from Hell that accomplished little except proving that Sharpies were permanent.

When there was no hope, I turned to that savior and demon of humankind: Google.

According to the first few search results, I had one last hope: toothpaste. "You really have to scrub," the comment said, "but it shouldn't remove the finish."

I grabbed the Sensodyne, the Colgate, and the Crest. And I scrubbed. For twenty minutes.

And it came off. Unlike the red wine stains on my teeth, which got worse after this incident.

In his book *Outliers*, Malcolm Gladwell discusses the 10,000-hour rule. According to research, it takes 10,000 hours to become an expert at something. Let's assume that parents actively mind their children for six hours a day (notice I didn't include time you stuck them in the wind-up swing in front of that *Baby Einstein* DVD). That means most parents don't become experts until their children are at least four years old. By that point, we've already messed them up pretty badly. Thank you for illuminating that depressing statistic, Mr. Gladwell.

Another area where I've invoked the 10,000-hour rule more successfully is in developing useless talents. One of them is singing "Amazing Grace" off key to various tunes, something I do every time I see monkeys on the back of a motorcycle. Another useless talent I possess is contorting my arms and sticking my head through them. A final one is sneezing like Donald Duck. I've clocked my 10,000 hours pretending I'm an asthmatic duck in a sailor suit. I started when I was twelve: there is no better way for a babysitter to disarm a child who is sobbing for her parents who've just left for seven hours to get drunk at their best friend's wedding. I'm pretty sure sneezing like Donald Duck could get me out of a traffic ticket.

Sneezing like Donald Duck ups my cool quotient with children under eight years old. If they're nine or older, though, sharing this talent becomes the Black Friday of my stock value.

My children frequently begged me to use my useless talent. Now I'm all for children begging their parents; it's the only way we get to feel like we're in control. If I refuse to sneeze like Donald Duck, they run around the house like a pair of wingless fowl in flu season.

 Parenting Tip: Train your children to beg; it will help you feel more in control than you actually are.

Like any good parent, I used my useless talent as leverage. "Mommy will sneeze like Donald Duck if you pick up your toys," I said. It was one of the few threats I made that I would carry through with, unlike the "If you don't pick up your toys, I'm going to put them all in the blender and make you drink them for breakfast."

I think I'll stick with Donald Duck's Center for Disease Control sound bite.

YOU DON'T NEED CLOTHES TO BE A DANCER

The best advice I ever got about parenting came from my older brother. "Don't be in a hurry to toilet train your kids."

This advice has come to underscore one of my theories of childrearing: If you wait long enough, your children will just do it themselves. It worked for breastfeeding; Vivian and William weaned themselves. Years later, I'd learn that it worked for tying shoes, riding bikes, and braiding hair.

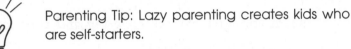

Parenting Tip: Lazy parenting creates kids who are self-starters.

My brother's advice worked for toilet training. By the age of three, William and Vivian just started to use the toilet themselves. No potty, no charts, no placing Cheerios or food coloring in the toilet bowl on purpose. Just a lazy mom who couldn't be arsed.

Getting rid of their pacifiers required a bit more ingenuity. Vivian and William had been sleeping with these plugs since they were tiny, and they'd developed the habits of long-term smokers, dangling their pacifiers out of their mouths like they were lit cigarettes, waving them around for emphasis when they were speaking, and frantically looking for another fix before bedtime. Since my ignore-and-they'll-figure-it-out approach was not working, I applied another one of my parenting strategies, which was also not in any books: I lied.

Parenting Tip: Lying is an invaluable strategy for parents. Start practicing as soon as you're pregnant.

It was autumn. Chris had volunteered to take over the gardening. He was cleaning up our flower beds by pulling all our perennials, which he thought were undercover weeds.

I, meanwhile, went to William and Vivian and told the most heart-wrenching fib I could create.

"I think it's time to get rid of your dummies," I said. We'd used the British euphemism for pacifiers since we'd lived in Thailand.

William and Vivian's eyes grew big and they searched their pockets for their addiction.

"There are other babies in the world who need dummies," I said, employing my best Sally-Struthers-help-underprivileged-children voice. "I think we should send them to Santa Claus." Four unblinking eyes stared at me. "Santa will deliver the dummies to other babies at Christmas."

Both Vivian and William looked down and nodded.

"For babies?" Will said.

I nodded.

"They won't cry," Vivian said.

I nodded again.

Those two little urchins went on a mass dummy sweep, searching for pacifiers that had been lost since dinosaurs walked the earth, which was the last time I'd vacuumed their room. William and Vivian found many amid dust bunnies and long forgotten library books. I grabbed a large envelope and addressed it to Santa. We deposited the dummies in it, and I threw it in the garbage when they weren't looking. The score: Made-Up Parenting 1; Parenting Books 0.

With their pacifiers in a landfill, we survived the night and the winter and spring. It was time to stir things up again, this time with a car trip.

William and Vivian became good car travelers early on, mostly because they were easily hypnotized by the hang-from-the-rafters DVD player in our minivan. Occasionally, though, guilt would set in and we'd stop the *Dora the Explorer* marathon. After we ignored them for long enough, Vivian and William would invent their own games. Sometimes it was I Spy; sometimes it was a game that had the same amount of logic as the parents of toddler beauty contestants competing on *Jeopardy*.

We were driving through Saskatchewan, which is like North Dakota, but with fewer people and straighter roads. The directions for driving across the Prairie Provinces are this: Drive in a straight line until you want to slit your wrists; you're 10 percent there. Every few hundred miles, there were signs along the highway that said, "Watch for pedestrians." I once asked Chris if there was a prize if we saw one.

We were in one of these long stretches when I noticed something was going on behind me. I craned my already spasm-ing neck. Vivian and William were wriggling and contorting themselves behind their blankets. I watched this for the length of three wheat fields until I figured it out.

"They're playing hide and seek," I said. "In their car seats."

Brilliant.

Maybe this was proof our children didn't qualify for early admission to Mensa. More likely it was proof that our DNA wouldn't fetch much at the cloning auction.

If you want to figure out which phrases you repeat over and over, have children. Then put them with you in a minivan for fifteen hours where you have to listen to them. According to my two little research blobs, I say "actually" and "God help me" all the time.

The various monologues I'd performed in front of William and Vivian all went something like this:

"Actually, if you could just clean up your toys." And when they didn't: "God help me."

"Actually, if you could stop biting your brother in the arm . . ." And when she didn't: "God help me."

"Actually, if you could just open that bottle of wine for me . . ." followed by "God help me."

It worked.

And my kids parroted it back to me.

Unfortunately, they also repeated what Chris said. We were driving Mile 462 on our cross-prairie, masochistic trip. Our twins were absorbed in the episode of *Dora the Explorer* where Dora couldn't find the object right in front of her so she yelled. We enjoyed a five-minute conversation, a full two minutes more than we talked the previous week.

Chris started telling me about what happened the previous day. "When I was driving the kids to the library yesterday morning, an A-hole passed me in a playground zone."

My mind sped up, wondering if Chris chose to "educate" this driver, his euphemism for giving the wrongdoer the finger and laying on the horn.

"So, I yelled out the window at him," he explained. "Then he sped past me."

God help me, I thought.

"But one block later," Chris continued, "Vivian asks me, 'Daddy, what does *bucking slow down* mean?'"

"You didn't say that in front of them, did you?" I asked.

"No, I *yelled* it," he said. "But I didn't think they heard it because I had Marilyn Manson cranked on the stereo."

At that point I realized why our kids didn't listen to us: Chris had ruined their hearing.

God help me.

Actually.

 Parenting tip: Having a father who is actively involved in childrearing will ensure kids learn street skills, like cursing.

Learning words like *bucking* is not the only advantage of having a dad who's actively involved with childrearing. They learned plenty, a fact I realized after our minivan clocked 832 miles and pulled into my parents' farmyard in Manitoba. My mom took the kids, and my dad got me a cold beer. It was good to be home.

We sat outside, enjoying the company of the nine billion mosquitoes even after slathering on DDT. "No one we know has contracted West Nile Virus this year," my mom said. The year the twins were born, my aunt and cousin had both been deathly ill with it. But that was distant history. So we let the kids run around.

I loved watching Vivian and William play on the farm. Their imagination went beyond suburban indoor games, where their only pursuits seemed to be "wrestling until someone bled" and "hop-on-mom until she puked." I wasn't sure who taught them either of these games, but it affirmed the *Lord of the Flies* theory of children: If you leave them be for too long, they will kill. Or at least devolve.

So we left them. It didn't hurt that my mom had brought some of my vintage Fisher Price people out to occupy the twins.

I had just finished telling Chris how I used to know how to open a beer bottle with a seat belt. He had just finished asking some suburban question, like, "Why didn't you just twist the cap off?" My parents sat proudly.

I heard barking, pretty convincing barking. This was not Fluffy the Dog, but Killer. We stopped our conversation. We heard this: "Good, Doggie. Good. Now sit."

We turned our attention to my kids. William sat obediently in front of Vivian, panting.

"Now fetch." Vivian flung a Fisher Price person, the angry, pissed-off boy in a cap. William crawled after it, retrieved it in his mouth, and deposited it in front of his master.

"Good, Doggie."

William barked.

"You know," I said, "human beings aren't supposed to bark or play fetch." I liked to ruin their fun whenever I got a chance.

Both kids looked at me with puppy dog eyes.

"OK, whatever," I added.

Parenting tip: Be the rain on your children's parade. This will help them to develop realistic outlooks on life.

I took a sip of my beer. The adult conversation progressed to the price of wheat.

That's when I heard it. Screaming. Not the fake kind. The someone-dropped-a-knife-on-me kind. I ran.

William held his arm.

Vivian hid in a shrub, crying.

"What happened?"

Will's screams subsided to sobs. "Vivian . . . bit . . . me."

"Vivian!" I said. "Did you bite him?"

She looked out from under the branches and nodded.

"Why?"

"We were playing doggie. Dogs bite."

I processed this for a minute. "But you were the owner."

When they weren't being dogs, William and Vivian loved to dance. A few times a week, we waltzed around the kitchen, jived in the entry, or crazy danced in the living room.

Vivian wished that we'd sign her up for dance classes. I knew there were a zillion benefits to dance, from coordination to confidence, but I couldn't deal with it. It was outside my comfort realm. We didn't dance on the farm.

I also didn't do hair. And I didn't do buns, unless there was a tasty sausage or burger in them. I didn't want to spend my free time watching YouTube videos to figure out how to do a hairstyle she had to wear. I also didn't do makeup on kids.

Plus, we knew what her gene pool contained: ballet wasn't in the picture, though speed skating was.

One afternoon, Vivian was trying on clothes from the ancient dress-up trunk in my parents' basement. She had just finished an impromptu dance recital at the farm. She started begging me to buy her special dance clothes: the tutu, the tights, the Lycra. I refused. She begged.

"Vivian," I explained, "you don't need clothes to be a dancer."

Vivian said something, but I missed it because Chris dropped the knife he was using to slice cheese for the burgers my dad was barbecuing.

Excellent. I have a double major in English and Women's Studies. I rant on the problem of sexualizing young girls, including bare midriffs, words on bums, and high heels. And now, I'd just told my daughter she could be a nude dancer.

Mommy needed a time out.

THE SAPPY FILES, PART 3 (OR WHY MY SON'S FUTURE THERAPISTS SHOULD ADORE HIM)

Dear William,

During the past year, you've mastered using manners to get what you want. You'd wander over, raise both of your hands like a referee signaling touchdown, and say, "May I please have some pick-me-up?"

"Yes," I'd say, putting aside whatever I was doing, "you may have some pick-me-up."

This phrase has become part of our family lore, one of those stories that I hope we'll always tell and that I hope you'll always love to hear.

Last week, we were at a dinner party with our friends, enjoying conversations with them and their worldly teen daughters.

"I want to go home," you said, ignoring social conventions that adults know too well.

"William, that's rude," I said and smiled apologetically at our hosts while helping myself to more wine.

You paused and tried again. "May I please have some go-home-now?"

You simultaneously broke my heart and made it stronger.

And then there's your delightful sneakiness. You've always been our night owl, staying awake long after Vivian (and sometimes Daddy) falls asleep. You read, sing, and sigh, twist in your blankets to find that magical spot. Lately, you've added escape artist to this nightly ritual.

On several occasions, you've grabbed your duvet, commando crawled past the bedroom where Daddy was, tiptoed down the stairs, and hid around the corner from where I sat under lamplight. I usually spotted your bare toes first.

"William?" I'd say.

"Mommy," you'd answer, stepping forward with your head down, pulling your duvet like Linus. "Can't sleep."

I'd look at you, trying to decide if I should send you back to your room or invite you to stay.

Usually, you'd make the decision for me.

"May I please have some up?" you'd ask. You knew that I could turn down neither good manners nor an extended hug. You were indeed an old soul, something my friend's mom noted about you when you were just months old.

I closed my laptop, placed it on the footstool, and made room for you, your blanket, and the finite number of cuddles I knew lay ahead.

Heart you always.

Much love,

Mommy

PART FOUR

PRESCHOOL, OR WHO TAUGHT YOU THAT?

EATING KIDS' HALLOWEEN CANDY IS A COMMUNITY SERVICE

For the first thirteen months of their Bangkok lives, Vivian and William wore socks once: for their Christmas trip home to winter wonderland. Living in a tropical country conditioned them to despise socks. Having sock-ist kids seems harmless. And it is, providing their toes don't turn black and fall off when they endure Canadian winters.

Failing to pick up discarded socks, however, is not harmless. My body knows this, because one moment I'm picking up sock number nine for the day, and the next moment I'm doing an octogenarian shuffle, one hand planted in the small of my back.

Vivian and William have an addiction to shedding socks. They start with a single pair, and end the day with multiple socks, passed out all over the house, strewn about, some in pairs, some alone, some in groups. By dinnertime, it looks like we've hosted a frat party.

Chris does laundry loads of socks, and he bribes the kids to put their clothes away. One day I did some math and calculated that 112 percent of the socks belong to William.

"Now that Will's in preschool, we need to help him kick his six-socks-a-day habit," I said.

Chris looked up from his iPhone and asked, "Do you think there's an app for that?"

Chris rarely criticizes me. I think he's learned it's pointless. Even when I leave twelve pairs of my shoes in our small entry or a knee-deep pile of clothes beside my bed, he lets it be. You can learn a lot from the way a person handles criticism. When he does dis me, I employ what he calls the Foghorn Leghorn approach. I ditch my rational brain and go into cartoon rooster mode. Disputes are settled with "You can't tell ME what to do. I'm gonna DO what I wants to DO."

 Parenting Tip: When you're arguing with your spouse over parenting issues, imitate a cartoon character to defuse the situation.

When Chris is criticized, he becomes silent, like a ticking bomb that needs to be defused.

Vivian goes into full-on, freak-out mode, eyes bulging like she stepped out of an episode of *The Simpsons*.

William reacts in his own way. He becomes Saving-Face Boy.

One day, William got tired of his sister stealing his favorite toy car, so he kicked her. Had her leg been a football, he would've scored a field goal.

"William!" I yelled. "No kicking your sister. Say you're sorry."

"No."

"William?" I growled.

"No."

"Then sit on the time-out chair until you're ready to say you're sorry."

He climbed into the armchair. Choosing the coziest chair as the time-out corner wasn't our smartest decision, but it does explain why I put myself in time out on a daily basis.

I comforted a crying Vivian, reprimanded her for stealing her brother's toys, and sent her upstairs to see Chris.

> Parenting Tip: Putting yourself in time-out is brilliant. Shackling yourself to the liquor cabinent is extra brilliant.

I went back to the kitchen to work my way through my least favorite Sisyphean task: unloading and loading the dishwasher. I was cursing at a knife stuck in the cutlery rack when someone tapped me. I turned around and saw William with a gigantic grin on his face. He was dressed upside down. In the place of his pants was his shirt; he'd stepped his legs into the shirtsleeves and was holding the shirt's waistband up to his belly button. On his head was his underwear.

"William," I said, "take the underwear off your head and put it back on your butt."

Saving-Face Boy smiled.

"And then go say sorry to your sister, OK?"

I picked up his pants and watched him waddle up the stairs in search of his sister.

Days later, after Vivian had taken a few tours of duty in the time-out chair, it was William's turn again. He sat there stoically while I prepared dinner, which involved measuring the water to boil macaroni in. When I had finished pouring in eight cups, I looked into the living room. William was nowhere to be found. Vivian, however, was relaxing in the time-out chair in an interesting outfit.

"William?" I called. "Come finish your time out."

Vivian answered. "It's OK, Mom. I sent him upstairs. I'm finishing his time out for him."

"You're finishing it? Did you volunteer for this job?"

"Yes," she said smiling.

"Interesting," I said, my automatic reply when I'm speechless or not listening.

Chris looked up from the newspaper, enjoying his night off from cooking. "Look out," he said, "they're starting to band together."

"I know," I said.

Then I turned my eyes to Vivian and the outfit she had changed into since arriving home from preschool. She was sashaying around the kitchen in black sparkly tights, a red sleeveless shirt she thought was a dress, and more bling than a rapper at a jewelry show.

She paraded towards the table, where I was trying to enjoy a late afternoon cup of tea before the Kraft Dinner water boiled. Vivian executed several catwalk turns but all I could notice was her lack of pants.

I must not have imbibed enough caffeine that day. I blurted, "You are not wearing that. My number one job is to keep you off the pole." I had burst her bubble.

"Don't I look beautiful?"

"You do, sweetie. You'd look beautiful in a paper bag. But you're not wearing that either. Not even for dinner."

Vivian paused. "What do you mean I can't go *on the pole?*"

At this point, Chris put down his newspaper. He smiled. "Not only did you steal that line from Chris Rock," he said, "but you have to explain yourself."

"Well, Vivian," I said, "if you wear clothes like that, you can't climb up the poles on the monkey bars because people will see your underwear. Please go change."

I got up, poured the Kraft Dinner out of the box into the eight cups of boiling water, and persuaded her to wear something less Gaga-ish. I could multitask when I had to.

"See?" I said to Chris. "I can steal and adapt."

The one time it's acceptable to dress like a skank is Halloween, God's gift to wannabe prostitutes. I suck at Halloween. I also suck at birthdays, Thanksgiving, and Easter. I do a half-arsed job with Christmas.

I approach most major holidays with a two-step strategy: (1) procrastinate, then (2) cram. Why shop ahead when stores are open December 23? Why buy a birthday gift when your husband purchased six Rubbermaid containers filled with LEGO at a garage sale last year? Why ask your children what they want to be for Halloween when you have twenty costumes in a trunk in the basement?

It's worked so far. What we save in money, we'll pay for in therapy.

Vivian and William were born under the Gemini sign, which makes them twins born under the sign of twins. How freaking unoriginal. According to the high science of astrology, my children display the following traits: they are versatile, lively, and responsive. Although these characteristics describe every child who isn't comatose, they are still fairly accurate descriptors of William and Vivian. Lively? Yes, just drop by my house at 6:00 AM any day, especially weekends. Versatile? Yes, if five-minute Jekyll to Hyde transformations can be evidence of that. They aren't usually responsive, unless they've consumed chocolate, and then they turn into Tasmanian Devils on Speed.

Tasmanian Devils on Speed are the mascots of Halloween, the holiday that lasts longer than merited. From picking up candy wrappers under the couch to refereeing wrestling matches over who owns the last bag of Doritos, Halloween creeps into November like a zombie elf.

Every year on October 30, I tell Vivian and William, "Go downstairs and find a costume." They get bonus candy if they choose an outfit that fits them and another if they choose one that accommodates a snowsuit.

William would be happy enough to trick-or-treat in his underwear with a towel around his neck: Super Boxer Boy. Vivian is a bit more work. But she gets bonus candy for creativity.

That particular Halloween, she went as an elephant ballerina. Yes, she added a pink tutu over the gray elephant costume. Before we ventured out into the near-winter temps, she danced for us.

"That is the best pirouette by a pachyderm I've ever seen," I said.

And it was.

The best part of Halloween is not the costumes, but the candy you can steal from children, preferably your own.

The day after Halloween, I placed the candy bowls on top of the fridge in the interests of controlling chocolate-induced misbehavior. This way, I could be the Queen of Candy Dispersal. This worked until my subjects staged a rebellion.

The Saturday following Halloween, while I attempted to sleep until seven, William and Vivian went downstairs for a snack. Normally, they'd grab an apple or a bagel but not this time.

When I awoke to silence, I trudged downstairs to find this scene: William stood on the cupboard, passed chocolates to Vivian who used scissors to remove the packaging. It was a streamlined assembly line that, if copied on a larger scale by North American automakers, would boost their productivity tenfold.

Judging by William and Vivian's chocolate-covered clown faces, they were enjoying the unionized coffee breaks.

I shut down that workplace fun and relished my role as foreman.

Later that night, after Vivian and William were passed out in a sugar coma, I revisited my plan. I saw my favorite, Reese's Peanut Butter Cups.

"Are you eating the kids' candy?" Chris asked.

"Hm-hmmm," I replied.

I chewed and then added, "Eating kids' Halloween candy is a community service."

He looked unconvinced so I continued.

"Seriously, they'll have fewer cavities and fewer fights. The community wins."

"No," he said. "You win."

"Of course I do. I am the community."

 Parenting Tip: To ensure your kids don't get cavities, eat as much of their Halloween candy as possible.

WE CAN USE THE MONEY FROM THE KIDS' ACCOUNT TO PAY THE CREDIT CARD BILL

Chris's parents volunteered to look after William and Vivian at our house that fall so Chris and I could jet off to Virginia where my close friend was getting married. It was our first time away from our kids, who were now four years old. We stayed in an old plantation mansion bed and breakfast, in the James Madison room. I remember because the portrait of President Madison was so lifelike, his eyes following me around the room, especially when I undressed. A hand towel covered the picture for the remainder of our stay.

While I was being ogled by President Madison in Orange County, Grandma and Grandpa were entertaining William and Vivian in suburbia. Chris's parents had come bearing their usual gifts: ten pounds of organic beef, homemade pierogi, and bags of loose change. This time they brought something else: a Snakes and Ladders game.

This was a problem.

I'd tried to introduce board games before. Checkers weren't successful, even with coaching. Vivian had a first-rate meltdown when her dad crowned his third king. This was the girl who felt slighted that her brother won the out-of-the-womb race. Since that day in 2004, she had to win. After she kicked the entire checker board, causing a black and white hailstorm, Chris remarked, "Now I know how Michael Jordan's parents felt."

When Chris's parents babysat so their son could shoot AK-47s in rural Virginia and so I could help the bride with wedding preparations by drinking margaritas, Grandpa decided to introduce his grandchildren to the timeless Snakes and Ladders game. I know because he recounted it to us several times when we returned. Usually through fits of laughter.

Grandpa took William into the living room with the game board and pieces. Grandpa explained the game, trying to get William to focus on the rules rather than classifying the venomous snakes. Grandpa started the game, listening to William spout a myriad of snake facts.

"Come on, William," he said. "Now it's your turn to throw the dice. Go on."

When Grandpa told this story, he always paused at this point.

With an invitation to throw the dice, William did just that. He launched the dice across the room with a fastball throw.

It took them fifteen minutes to find both dice. I was onto my second margarita in that same time frame.

I had, however, experienced dice throwing on my own. During a weak moment when I decided to try to parent we tried Clue Junior. This is the script from our first game:

> Vivian: "I made a mistake, I get to go again, it's not fair, I didn't mean to!" Tears welled up in her eyes.
>
> William: "If she goes again, she's cheating." He threw the die.
>
> Me: "Let's stop and call it a tie." I pick up the game pieces, including the die in the adjacent room.
>
> William: "I never win. No one loves me." He exited to weep on the staircase.
>
> Vivian: "Let's sell this game." She stepped over her brother, stomped upstairs, slammed the bedroom door.

Vivian's idea was one possibility: sell all the games. Another one was to hire a babysitter and go out without the kids.

Going to Virginia was a one-off trip. Chris and I had hired babysitters for a couple hours, but that was infrequent. This disappointed our twins. They'd always loved the scant time they'd had with babysitters, even if Vivian and William didn't always understand the job description.

When Vivian was a toddler, she asked, "Mom, do babysitters sit on babies?"

I asked her to repeat herself. I tended to tune out my children until I sensed there was some substance in their comment.

 Parenting Tip: Develop selective listening skills. Practice on your spouse.

Vivian repeated herself.

"No," I said, "babysitters don't actually sit on babies." I paused. "Has your babysitter ever sat on you?"

Vivian laughed. "No," she said. "But why are they called babysitters?"

I gave her a nine-minute lecture on etymology and root words. She left after the second minute.

I was confident that Vivian and William's babysitter not only never sat on them, but also never lectured them. Because they adored her. I had a few theories on why they loved having other people look after them.

Theory One had to do with the fact that William and Vivian are twins. There was comfort in numbers, especially when your partner-in-crime had been with you since the womb. It also couldn't hurt when you outnumbered your babysitter 2:1. Odds like this increased the chance that you were running the family enterprise, especially when the CEO and CFO were AWOL.

Theory Two as to why our kids loved babysitters was because William and Vivian spent their first year in Thailand. It all went back to the Coca-Cola deliveryman, waitresses, and drunken women cuddling our twins.

Theory Three as to why our kids adored babysitters was that we were lousy parents. We no longer read parenting books bettering ourselves nor had we ever carved pumpkins with them. We were just kind of there. We once took Vivian and William sledding on New Year's Day, and that was pretty much the Event of Their Lives. I figured if you set the bar low, it was easy to maintain the standard. Needless to say, when they had a babysitter, the endless games of hide and seek and make-believe fueled their love for their babysitter and provided a foil for our lackluster parenting.

 Parenting Tip: Dare to be lousy parents; your children will love having babysitters, which means you'll go out more frequently.

One Saturday morning, my twins plotted in a corner, eventually sending Vivian to me as an envoy.

"Mom," she said, "we haven't seen our babysitter in a while."

"That's because Daddy and I haven't gone out in a while."

Vivian paused, looking back to William who was eavesdropping. "Can you guys go out?" she asked.

I took her hint, called our babysitter, and informed Chris of our evening plans.

The rest of the day passed slowly, as it often does when you have children.

William broke the silence that didn't exist. "How long until she comes?"

I looked at my watch. "Fifteen minutes."

"Fifteen minutes?" William repeated. He gazed out our picture window, eyes big. "But, Mom, it's really dark outside."

Tears streamed down his cheek. I knelt down, eye level with my now-sobbing son. Vivian came and rubbed his back. William rarely wept, so when he did, we assumed roles as investigators and psychologists.

"What's wrong, William?" I asked.

"It's, it's, it's . . . dark out."

I wiped his tears away.

"Mommy and Daddy won't be gone long. We'll be home soon. Just after you fall asleep."

"Fifteen minutes is a long time," William said. "What if she doesn't come?"

Epiphany.

"Are you worried your babysitter won't come?"

"Yes."

"Then you're not upset because you want Mommy and Daddy to stay home with you?"

"No." He looked up and wiped his snotty nose on my sleeve. "I just want her to come right now."

All that crying over the fear he was going to be stuck with his mommy and daddy.

Minutes later, the doorbell rang, easing his fears. Before I could remind the babysitter where the lifetime supply of Band-Aids was or the phone number for 9-1-1, the kids had begun a raucous game of tag with their babysitter chasing them around the house.

Hiring our babysitter over the Christmas season helped escalate the financial strain of the holiday. Why everyone has to throw a party in December instead of a boring month like February mystifies me.

Even though I despised shopping, I loved Christmas. It wasn't the presents, the word *naughty*, or the eggnog; it was Santa. Now I may have had a thing for men in uniforms and facial hair, but Santa was more than that. At Christmas time, our Santa-fied society encouraged me to lie to my children, something I did all the time. Only now I did it guilt free.

Once November came, I used the Santa card. Whenever Vivian and William fought, like they did numerous times during their preschool astrophysics unit on the solar system, I said one word: "Santa."

So there I was, sitting in the living room, drinking tea with a friend while Norah Jones crooned on the stereo. This peaceful tableau lasted about five minutes before being interrupted by murderous screams.

I climbed the stairs in three strides and started with my usual parenting question: "Hey, hey, what's going on here?"

"He's hitting me," Vivian screamed.

"She hit me first," William countered.

The tennis game continued, with blame being volleyed over the net with surprising endurance. Then the time out, a metaphorical one, when I attempted to figure out what the real problem was.

"William says there's lava on Neptune," Vivian shouted.

"Lava?"

"I mean fire," said Will.

"Fire?"

"Yes."

"There's no fire on Neptune," Vivian said.

"Yes there is."

"No there's not."

"Stop!" I shouted.

I resolved this with one word: Santa.

Later, after my friend had fled the scene, more interplanetary warfare came my way.

With both kids safely tucked in, I curled up on the couch and watched *It's a Wonderful Life*. Somewhere during one of

Clarence's sermons, the screaming started again. This time Vivian and William yelled and wrestled their way downstairs.

"Mom," asked Vivian, "what's the hottest planet?"

"Umm, I don't know—Mercury?"

"See, I told you so," said Vivian.

"No it's not. It's Venus," said William.

"Well, Mercury is the closest," I added, proud that I knew one scientific fact.

"But Venus is hotter."

"No it's not."

"OK, OK. I'm calling Santa," I said.

"Does he know a lot about the planets?"

"I don't know," I said. "But he'll care that you're arguing and being naughty."

Both kids wandered up to bed, defeated by the mere mention of a fictional man in a red suit.

The next night, both kids rushed into our bedroom to inform us that Pluto sometimes orbited closer to Earth than Neptune.

I preempted them. "If you're going to fight about this, I'm calling Santa."

Will shuffled his feet. "Has he started learning about the planets?"

"Maybe."

"Will he even answer your call?" Vivian asked.

"What?"

"Well, isn't he too busy to talk to you?"

I looked at Chris. "Trust me," I said. "Santa always takes my calls. Now go to bed. Enough planets." They left, pushing each other all the way to their room.

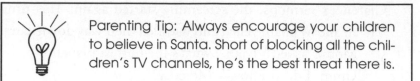

Parenting Tip: Always encourage your children to believe in Santa. Short of blocking all the children's TV channels, he's the best threat there is.

I turned off the TV.

"Where are you going?" asked Chris.

"To prepare for tomorrow's fight, which I'm guessing will be 'Is Pluto really a planet?'"

"Don't bother," he said. "They're in agreement on that one. They call it a dwarf planet."

"Isn't that a little person planet?" I asked.

Chris smiled. "Come back here. Let's watch Jimmy Stewart. I brought the DVD upstairs," he said.

Christmas came, as did Santa. Chris, William, and Vivian were impressed I knew how to make waffles that didn't come in a box.

"You should make these every morning," William said.

I nodded. "Right."

This was why I taught full time. It was easier to get ninety-seven teens to listen than it was my own children.

Unfortunately, Santa didn't bring debt relief. We had limited income and were not one of those fiscally organized families. Some people were careful: they had savings accounts for emergencies. Some people were careless: they had children.

Apparently when one drives a vehicle—even if it's a minivan—the ability to brake is important. Apparently when one's brakes start squealing, it means the brake pads are worn through and are now wrecking the brake drums. Hello, credit card.

Five days later, our financial problems heated up when the hot water heater in our basement died.

Then, our garage door came off its hinges, warped, and ceased functioning.

I began to think my brain was sending an electromagnetic force field that would cause expensive things to malfunction.

The credit card bill came. Thousands. My electromagnetic force field had a meltdown.

We couldn't afford thousands.

"What are we going to do?" I asked Chris.

"Pay it off eventually," he said.

"At twenty percent interest?" I asked.

We sat in silence.

"I have an idea," I said.

He looked up.

"We can use the money from the kids' account to pay the credit card bill."

"You're serious?" Chris asked.

"Why not? We'll put it back. Some day."

DID YOU PEE ON MINNIE MOUSE ON PURPOSE?

I'm not one of those moms who is psycho about cleanliness. I believe that the best proof that kids are kids is if they're dirty, just like the best proof politicians are politicians is if they're dirty.

 Parenting Tip: If your kids are dirty, it means they're building up their immunity. Screw nightly baths.

When William and Vivian were babes, we bathed them daily. This torturous ritual was necessary due to Bangkok's heat and the curdled milk that started to stink in the creases of our babies' fat.

Once we returned to the land of winter, daily baths were history, as was disposable income, pedicures, and prostitutes offering Chris sexual favors for $5 when he walked to the supermarket.

Some of these changes were good.

William, however, became accustomed to not washing his hair. Every week or so, I'd insist on washing it, especially with him in preschool. I thrived on appearing like I was a half decent parent.

Will often protested. One time I made the mistake of reasoning with him.

"If you don't wash your hair," I said, "things will start growing in it."

William stopped playing with his shark toy. "Like vegetables?"

I laughed. "Well, maybe not vegetables. But bugs. Oil." I paused. "And yes, vegetables. You don't want broccoli growing out of your head, do you?"

"No," he said. "I don't even want carrots."

Eventually he got out of the bath, and eventually Chris and I took Vivian and William on errands.

The mercury had dipped to minus fifteen. I was trying to get my two abominable-looking children herded into our minivan while Chris scraped the windshield. Then, it happened. Like a car crash in slow motion, William approached the van's frosty sliding door with his tongue. It didn't matter that the van hadn't been washed since 2002. People like us could be one of the reasons Canada has a large supply of fresh water.

I watched. In short quick tongue-lashings, William started to enjoy a frost-covered van.

"William? Stop."

Before I could find more words, Vivian mimicked him and enjoyed her own mixture of the winter triumvirate: dirt, salt, and frost.

Finally, my brain communicated with my tongue. "For crying out loud," I said. "Don't lick the minivan. Your tongue could fall off."

They looked at me like I was stupid or lying.

"Really. When I was a kid, I licked the monkey bars at school and my tongue got stuck."

What I didn't know was that Chris was listening. "You licked the monkey bars?" he asked.

"Yes. And my tongue got stuck."

"I imagine it did," he said. I could see his breath as he laughed.

"It wasn't funny," I said.

"It is now."

"I don't make fun of you for going to School Patrol Camp."

"Yes, you do."

"Was it really a sleep away camp?" I asked.

"Time to get inside the van, kids. You too, Lee."

We finished our errands and returned to our warm house, where the ratio of stuffed animals to people was 106:4. If any of my kids' stuffed animals had a pulse, the SPCA would be on us in a second. As it was, we were lying low from the producers of hoarder reality shows.

Very few of the stuffed animals in our menagerie were purchased new. Fewer still were washed. This meant we provided shelter for several dozen stuffed animals carrying diseases.

Most of these stuffed animals were named. William and Vivian used to say night-night to each of them. It was our own endless version of *Goodnight Moon*.

We had stuffies whose names were based on appearance (Rainbow Bear), stuffies named after strippers (Roxy), and stuffies that revealed our kids' hearing defects, like Little Pusky, the husky dog.

Then we had Minnie Mouse. How un-freaking-original. Chris wanted us to be a Disney-free house, but that declaration lasted about as long as my plan not to use a TV as a babysitter. Could I put Baby Einstein on repeat play before my kids were one? You bet.

Minnie Mouse featured prominently in a catastrophe when Vivian and William were stuck inside because it was minus thirty outside. Vivian, the owner of the beloved mouse in a polka dot dress, came and told me her favorite stuffy of the day was soaked. Some basic detective work told me the smell wasn't water.

It was then that I strung together a series of words that I am certain have never been uttered in the history of the English language: "Who peed on Minnie Mouse?"

By now, Vivian had reverted to the fetal position and was sobbing.

"William? Did you pee on Minnie Mouse?"

"Yes, Mom," he said. "Sorry."

"Did you pee on Minnie Mouse on purpose or by accident?" Another series of words that have never been said.

"On purpose."

"Why?" I tried to ignore Vivian, now in full freak out mode, rather legitimately this time.

William shrugged.

My question remained unanswered.

A small miracle perhaps.

YOU CAN BUY A BABY AT THE HOSPITAL

A frequent question I get asked is "Do your twins get along?"

As with most twin questions, there are many answers to this. If I'm annoyed, I say, "Sometimes." If I'm in a rush, I say, "Yes." And if I feel like chatting, I say, "Like an old married couple."

It might be a weird comparison, but William and Vivian do remind me of an old married couple. Here's how:

- They're not outwardly smitten, but there's a quiet (and a not-so-quiet) sense of togetherness.
- They yell at each other when they retell the same old story.
- They make each other laugh in a way no other human can.
- They know precisely what annoys each other and are willing to twist that knife.
- They blame each other for their own errors.
- They burp and fart in front of each other.

That's enough warm fuzzies for one book.

During a two-week preschool Spring Break, however, Vivian and William spent more time together then they were accustomed to. At school, they were in separate all-day classes, so they were getting used to being apart. Or at least that was my theory.

So, like an old married couple that's seen no one but each other for two weeks, the annoyance levels ratcheted up.

It was William who was most vocal about this.

First, he told his sister, "I'm not inviting you to my birthday party." Vivian realized the implication of this as a twin and burst into sobs.

"William!" I chastised him. "You can't tell your twin sister she's not invited to your birthday."

The next day, he told her, "Give me my car back, or I'll throw you outside." Then he farted. Vivian farted back.

William's annoyance at too much together time continued. After uninviting her to his birthday party, he announced, "I want to sell Vivian." The first day he said this, I ignored it. Then, like a wart on the bottom of your foot, it remained a nuisance the next day.

"We can't sell your sister," I said.

"Why not?" he asked.

"Well, it's illegal, for one."

"I want to sell her anyway."

"It's mean."

"So?"

"William!"

"I want to sell her."

Logic wasn't working, so I employed a different strategy.

"Look," I said. "No one would buy her. You know that."

And he wandered away and found his LEGO. Silently.

So do they get along?

Sometimes.

For a full year, Vivian proclaimed her undying love for her classmate. It was mutual and they had worked out the living arrangements: after they graduated from high school, he was to move in with us. We'd met with the parents, and we were content with the situation. Once you have kids, arranged marriages make a lot more sense. Mind you, once you have kids, boarding school makes a lot more sense. As does birth control.

I have a theory that most interesting conversations happen in a motorized vehicle or in a canoe. Like most of my theories, this one is a fact.

On a springtime drive to preschool, William announced that he wanted to marry me.

Vivian, who's had this conversation before, said, "You can't marry your mom."

Without missing a beat, William said, "Then I'll marry Dad."

Vivian proceeded to educate her brother. "You can marry a guy, but you can't marry your dad. Or anyone in your family."

"Yup, she's right," I said. "You can't marry your sister . . . or me . . . or even your dad."

William sighed.

"Don't worry," I added. "You don't have to get married. And even if you want to get married, you have to be at least thirty."

Another one of my theories that I tried to pass off as fact.

I nearly revisited this topic when William and I played Superheroes, which involved making up your own superhero name and superpower. William didn't like it when I selected the name Miss Piggy or chose the superpower of being wealthy, so I was forced to be creative. I christened myself IncrediMommy who had the power to make everyone listen to her. This worked better than my other invented superhero: MegaLegga. Her superpower was that her feet were guns. To shoot, she had to stand on one leg in some unstable pose and wait for bullets to fire from the soles of her feet. William quickly figured out that he could duck under my shooting leg and push it toward the ceiling so I resembled a pretzel-ish can-can dancer. If he pushed hard enough on that high-kick leg, I'd fall on my butt and start wheezing and writhing on the ceramic tile floor. It was a fun game. For him.

Sometimes the game of Superheroes morphed into something more specific, like Tarzan. William would be Tarzan, and I'd be his sidekick James. I liked James. He just followed Tarzan around like a puppy waiting to be ordered around and possibly kicked. James swung on pretend vines, climbed trees, and brought Tarzan glasses of chocolate milk.

One day, I didn't feel like playing anything.

"Please, Mom?" he begged. "I need you to be James."

"I don't feel like it," I answered. "Plus, it's Tarzan and Jane, not Tarzan and James."

"No it's not. It's James."

"It's Jane, William. A girl's name."

With the look on his face, you'd have thought I told him that Diego had been torn limb from limb by Dora.

"I like James better," he said.

"I know, Sweetie."

"Jane's a girl."

"Yes, she is. But so are IncrediMommy and MegaLegga."

"Can James be Jane's twin?"

"Sure," I said.

"Can Jane stay home?"

"Yup. She sure can. She could use some time alone."

Vivian's questions didn't involve superheroes or marriage, but were more dangerous since they were about reproduction. I'm one of those parents who will give an honest answer to biological questions, but who also tells way too much. If my kids ask me about candy, I'll volunteer information about root canals. If my kids ask me about rugby, I'll end up describing the cannibal scene in the movie *Alive*. I'm pretty skilled at taking a banal topic and having it enter the difficult-to-talk-about realm.

So when Vivian asked about babies, I told her about vaginal births, C-sections, epidurals, placentas, and adoption.

William, of course, started out listening, but his Y-chromosome wiggled so he wandered away to partake in his own creation ritual: build, destroy, repeat.

Stereotypically, Vivian and I stood in the kitchen and spoke about all things birth related, rendering my degree in Women's Studies useless.

"Do I have to have a baby?" Vivian asked.

"No, Sweetie," I said.

"But I want a baby."

"Then you can have one."

"But I don't want to get it out."

"Trust me," I said. "After nine months, you'll want it out."

"But I don't want to have a baby come out of my vagina."

"I understand that."

"And I don't want the doctors to cut me with a knife to take the baby out."

"I understand that too. They do give you medicine."

"Is it by needle?"

"More or less."

"I hate needles."

"Well, you likely . . . Um . . . why don't we—"

We were interrupted by an epic crash in the living room. A Tarzan yell erupted and William started to hurl the remaining blocks at the windows and walls. Evidently I wasn't the only one stumbling and flailing.

"Can I just buy one at the hospital?" Vivian asked.

I rewound the tape in my brain, trying to recall our conversation.

"Great idea." I said, seeing a way out. "You can buy a baby at the hospital. When you're thirty."

Parenting Tip: To entertain your children, give them way too much information when they ask a question, especially if it involves explaining where babies come from.

IT'S NOT AN ICE CREAM TRUCK, IT'S A VEGETABLE TRUCK

I don't make hot breakfasts unless they're for Christmas dinnner; I don't change dishtowels until they walk to the washing machine on their own; and I don't do laundry.

I'd fail as a 1950s housewife, or as a 2010s one. This has impacted my children's vocabulary. Sure, they know some new words that I didn't as a child: Internet, Twitter, time out, girls night out, sarcastic, and margarita, but they also don't know some basic household words, including iron.

I had a weak moment that spring and let my children do a craft. Someone, who's now in the Witness Protection Program, gave William and Vivian a lifetime supply of Perler beads. If you don't know what these are, you've won the lottery. Put down this book and do a happy dance. Essentially, they are miniature plastic beads that will assault your vacuum for the next four years. They're also something little kids could choke on, but if you don't bother to read the fine print, you'd never know that.

Parenting Tip: Even lazy parents will occasionally let their child do a craft. Keep such moments of weakness to a minimum.

Still, I let my children attempt this Perler bead craft. God knows I couldn't help them with it; I have the finger dexterity of Kermit the Frog.

Anyway, I was on standby vacuum alert, sucking up the Perler beads when they hit the floor. When Vivian and William finished, I had to iron their creations in order to melt the plastic pieces into a beautiful glob.

After an impromptu scavenger hunt, I discovered the ironing board. It was making out in the back of a closet with the bread maker. When I found the actual iron, William asked, "What's that?"

I looked at him. "Are you serious?"

He nodded.

"Vivian," I said, "do you know what this is?"

"No."

"It's called an iron."

"What does it do?"

"Well, it takes wrinkles out of clothes. Grandma uses one."

Of course, Grandma also used window cleaner, Mason jars, and Bundt pans, none of which my children knew either.

One word William and Vivian did learn early was ketchup. It is an undisputed, unproven fact that 207 percent of children would not get their daily fruit and vegetable servings were it not for ketchup.

 Parenting Tip: If you count ketchup as a fruit or vegetable, it's likely your child is eating a balanced diet.

Now, some nutritionists might say that ketchup should not be included in the food pyramid. To them, I say go wild: have unprotected sex and see what happens when your offspring spits out a real tomato. If human experimentation is not their thing, I invite them to borrow my children for six months. By the end of those 729 days of babysitting, not only will ketchup be on the pyramid, but mayonnaise will be a protein, and chocolate-covered raisins and Cheez Whiz will be milk products.

William has put ketchup on everything, from pancakes to his sister. I think it's his version of peanut butter. I am a peanut butter nut. I put it on bananas, chocolate, ice cream, and apples. Ever since I saw my dad adding salt to a peanut butter sandwich, I realized it was the world's most versatile food. Unless you're allergic.

But back to William. On this particular day he ate ketchup on his rib eye steak, a heinous act that the beef lobby is petitioning Washington to make a crime in forty-seven states. Actually, William was not so much eating steak with ketchup as he was eating ketchup with a side of steak. Because William tended to eat in layers, saving the best for last, his steak disappeared faster than bad investments.

And then he went into efficiency mode, licking the plate of ketchup.

"William," I said. "Please use a fork to eat the ketchup."

I mean seriously. We were raising these children to have manners.

We were also raising them to see vegetables as a deterrent, another strategy that has yet to be the subject of a parenting book.

In the summer, the loudest sounds in our suburb are garage doors humming closed, lawn mowers sparking to life, and the occasional ice cream truck. Nothing like using the distorted sound of "It's a Small World After All" as an impetus for lying to your children.

Whenever the ice cream truck circled our neighborhood, William and Vivian would ask what that sound was. Each time, we answered the same: "It's the vegetable truck." We first uttered this refrain when our twins were two.

By the time they were in preschool, they'd announce, "The vegetable truck's coming." Then they'd continue playing, unmoved by the thought of door-to-door turnips.

 Parenting Tip: Never tell your child that the ice cream truck sells ice cream. Tell them it sells vegetables.

"Mom, the vegetable truck's stopping," Vivian said. She and William opened our back door and climbed onto the patio table, giving them a direct view over our fence. If you remember the sitcom *Home Improvement*, think Wilson on stilts.

"Jenna's getting vegetables," William announced. Now that our twins were nearly five, they were extra curious.

I watched Jenna, our neighbor, disappear behind the truck.

A moment passed. My lie hung in the summer air.

The ice cream truck and its ditty started up the street.

Jenna walked down the sidewalk, ice cream in hand.

Vivian and William muttered to each other before screaming, "Mom!"

I tried to perpetuate the lie. "Jenna's eating frozen broccoli. Really. It's not an ice cream truck. It's a vegetable truck."

"Then why is there a picture of ice cream on the truck?"

The myth disappeared faster than the jingle.

Add this to the list of things William and Vivian can tell their therapists in a decade.

HOP ON POP, IF YOU KNOW WHAT I MEAN

The month of May brought with it many things: my husband's birthday, which usually fell on Mother's Day, something nearly as unfair as child slavery; mosquitoes; and the birthday of my twins. It was the latter that caused me stress. If Monty Hall offered me three doors, where number one was lunch with Martha Stewart, number two was a dengue fever convention, and number three was a kids' birthday party, I'd choose the Psych Ward. At least they'd have good meds.

Not only was Vivian a child who asked a lot of questions, she was also a kid who could spot if you weren't listening. I could not get away with using fillers like "really," "uh-huh," or "interesting" while my mind thought of important items like how Colin Firth would sound saying my name with his yummy accent.

"Mom? Mom!" she said. "You're not listening to me."

"Yes, I am. You were saying something about Max. Or Ruby. Or their absent parents."

"No, I wasn't. I was talking about mosquitoes."

"Well, they both can be annoying," I said, starting to chop carrots for chili that my kids wouldn't eat.

"Mom!"

"OK, I'll listen this time," I said, shelving my Kingdom of Firthdom until bedtime.

"Do you know mosquitoes only live for a few days?"

"Yes, I do know that."

"Do you think they have birthday parties?" Vivian asked.

I stopped chopping and looked for part of my thumbnail among the carrot bits. "Nope. No birthday parties," I said.

"Are you sure?"

I threw the bit of nail that I found onto the floor and shoved the carrots into the Crock-Pot—or crock of pot, as it was called in our house.

"Yes," I said. "I'm absolutely certain mosquitoes don't have birthday parties. They don't even live for a year. How would they have a birthday party?"

"Their mommy could throw one for them," Vivian said. "They could have one every day since they don't live long."

"Their poor mom," I muttered, giving the chili a stir.

"Why is she poor?" Vivian asked.

"Because she lays hundreds of eggs in her lifetime. That'd be a lot of parties to plan."

I started to unpack the dishwasher. Vivian followed. If she were a mosquito, she'd be hovering.

"Mom?" she asked. "What are we doing for our birthday?"

"Waiting till we go see Grandma and Grandpa in July to celebrate it?"

"No, I want a party. Everyone has a party in preschool."

I walked around her to put away the knives. She was right. Every classmate did have a party, all organized by Martha Stewart.

"We'll have a party," I said. "Here. It's cheaper."

"Can we get a clown?"

"No."

"Why not?"

"Because there are two types of people in this world— people who hate clowns, and clowns."

"Don't say *hate*, Mom."

"Sorry."

"But why no clowns?"

"I'm scared of them."

"Really?"

"Yes."

"What about a magician?" she asked. "Are you scared of them?"

"Sometimes."

"Why?"

"They might make Mommy disappear." I paused, contemplating that delightful possibility. Then I frisbee-d Tupperware lids into a cupboard.

"No they won't," Vivian said. "They just make things disappear. Like money."

"My point exactly," I said. "Look, Vivian. No entertainment. Just good ol' fashioned fun and play." I thought back to my childhood parties, which consisted of playing with a couple of cousins in the basement while my aunts and uncles drank beer with my parents around the kitchen table.

"Can we at least have a cake?" Vivian asked.

"Yes, I can manage a cake," I said. "But just one. You're going to share it."

Off she ran to tell William about how she had worn down Mommy and they were having the first actual birthday party of their lives.

The next week, I emailed invites and discussed party plans with my husband.

"I don't do kids' parties," Chris said.

"You what?" I asked.

"I don't do birthday parties. I'm not going to be here."

"That's not fair."

"You're right," he said. "It's not. But I've got a work thing."

"No, you don't. It's not on the calendar. You put everything on the calendar."

"It's a *top secret* work thing."

"Isn't that in our vows?"

"The top secret work thing?"

"No," I said. "That both parents have to attend the birthday party. It's the in-sickness part. I'm sure."

"Sorry," he said.

"You realize you're going to pay for this."

Chris shrugged. "I'll help before and after. I just won't be here for the party. I have lots of stuff for birthday parties that I picked up at garage sales. You'll hardly need to do a thing."

The day before the party, I had to take William to another birthday party. Chris was out with Vivian buying more crap at garage sales that we could fill loot bags with.

I'm not sure who opts to have a birthday party for a horde of five year olds at a pool. The parents have to stay, don bathing suits, and try to prevent their offspring from going all goldfish-belly-up in the pool.

I wore my suck-everything-in, push-everything-up swimsuit that didn't manage to hide my thighs. William didn't seem to care. We waded in. I looked around. No one but dads. Evidently moms didn't want to get into bathing suits. William clung to me like I was the *Titanic* before it sank.

After discussing the NHL playoffs with a few uber-fans, William and I floated away to an even shallower area. He went down a slide and snorted chlorine.

Another dad came over. I watched his son do some pre-Olympic flip turns.

William sensed competition. He waded over. And blew his nose.

"You can't blow your nose in the pool," I said.

The dad mumbled something, backed away, and went to help his son perfect his butterfly stroke.

After the pool snot-fest, I picked up Vivian and dragged both my kids to the supermarket to buy food for their own birthday party, which was less than twenty-four hours away. I knew, because Vivian and William were showcasing their math skills by counting down. We picked up the prerequisite case of juice boxes, the vegetable tray that no one would eat, and a case of Band-Aids.

 Parenting Tip: Keep an emergency vegetable tray in the fridge. If other parents visit your home, pull it out and appear responsible.

Then they saw them. Balloons. The helium filled ones.

"Can we, Mom?"

"Please?"

"It's our birthday."

"Please, Mom."

I sighed. "Go ahead," I said. "One each. But only the cheap round ones."

They stared at the balloons longer than most men look at engagement rings.

"Hurry up," I said.

"I want this one," Vivian said. She pointed to a pink balloon that said HAPPY BIRTHDAY. I untangled it and tied it around her wrist.

I looked at William. "Come on, Will," I said. "Choose one."

"This one," he said, smiling.

I looked up and saw him pointing to a balloon with "65" on it. "The one that says sixty-five?" I asked.

William nodded.

"Why do you want that one?"

"Because next year I'm going to be six, and tomorrow I'm five."

We made it home with the balloons. Sometime while I was unpacking the groceries, William discovered he could attach the balloon to his remote control car and bang it into my ankles repeatedly. Vivian, meanwhile, occupied herself with a gift sent by her grandparents, a stick-on mosaic butterfly. This craft could be training for bomb disposal technicians. If it were me, I would have chucked the craft across the room after ten minutes of attempting to maneuver my barely opposable thumbs. She finished. She played with LEGO figurines for a bit, before I sent her and William upstairs with their balloons to spend time with their other mother, the TV.

Chris, who had yet to flee, pulled out nine boxes of kids' party supplies from the garage. He was pulling out stuff for loot bags and blowing off the dust.

"I'm not helping you do this, you know," I said.

"I know."

We did our respective chores in silence. In a rare moment of clarity, I realized the whole house was quiet. Too quiet. I climbed the stairs, but stopped at our landing. Lying there, in a Mattel crime scene, was a decapitated Ken doll. His head had rolled to the right of his body. Barbie lay nearby, motionless, with all body parts intact.

"Chris?" I called. "Someone decapitated Ken doll."

He walked over, anxious to put his CSI skills to the test. "He looks a lot like Stephen Harper," Chris said, looking at the head.

I smiled, wondering how many times Canada's Prime Minister had been compared to Ken doll.

I continued up the stairs and chastised the kids for drawing on their bedroom walls.

I managed to bake a pathetic-looking cake, clean the house, and think some more about Colin Firth. I bet he never made his beautiful Italian wife throw a birthday party.

The day arrived and, true to his word, Chris's flight impulse was activated. Shortly after he fled, the doorbell started ringing. Kids came. And so did parents.

Parents were staying? I hadn't counted on this. I thought every parent viewed birthday parties as I did: a chance to drop your kid off and get two hours of free time.

Nope. Some came in.

I made tea for the parents and started applying face paint to the children's faces.

If you can't draw a circle with a compass, don't even attempt to paint the face of a child. I attempted skulls on the boys' cheeks and pink hearts on the girls.

Somehow, time passed. We played pin the tail on the donkey, musical chairs, and every other childhood game I could think of. We opened gifts and had cake.

We waved as everyone left.

Chris returned four minutes later.

"How was it?" he asked.

I rolled my eyes.

Chris hugged both Vivian and William. "What happened to their cheeks?" he asked.

I growled. "Into the bath," I told the kids. "And wash that stuff off."

Chris cleaned up. I sat, guilt free.

After finishing her bath, Vivian pranced down the stairs in her robe. "What's that on your cheek?" I asked.

She felt her cheek.

"Come here," I said.

I looked at the red, pimply skin that was heart-shaped.

"I think you're allergic to the face paint," I said.

The next day, I picked Vivian and William up after school. They skipped to the minivan, climbed in, and told me about their school birthday party. I drove as they chatted. I stopped at a crosswalk in the parking lot to let a little girl and her mom pass. After they crossed, she turned around and waved. I saw a red heart shaped rash on her cheek.

My stomach sunk.

"Vivian," I asked, panicking. "Did any other girls have rashes from the face paint?"

"They all did, Mommy," she said. "We had matching hearts all day."

I drove home in a panic.

"Chris?" I called as I walked in the door. "The pink face paint gave all the girls rashes." I started to hyperventilate.

He started to laugh.

"It's not funny," I said, looking around for a paper bag.

"It kind of is," he said.

"Was the paint from a garage sale?" I asked.

"Of course."

"Was it used?"

"No. It was unopened. It's just old."

"@#$%! I infected a bunch of girls with tainted face paint. I can't believe it."

I headed to my computer. A quick search revealed headlines such as "FDA Issues Face Paint Warning," "Face Paint Can Have a Scary Side," and "Face Paint Recall."

I scanned the articles looking for words like "permanent scarring," "facial deformities," and "plastic surgery."

"Are you going to email the kids' parents?" Chris asked.

"Are you kidding?" I asked. "No way. That'll just instill fear in an already phobic population. Plus, the article says there are no long lasting side effects. So far."

Chris nodded.

"Look," I said. "Feel free to email them yourself. Explain where you bought the face paint."

"That's all right," he said. "The worst case scenario is that fewer people will come to Vivian and Will's birthday party next year."

Things were looking up.

Parenting Tip: Avoid purchasing second-hand face paint. If you do, use it only on your own children. This will limit the spread of infections. And don't even consider third-hand.

"Mom." Vivian stormed downstairs. "William won't let me watch any of my shows on TV. All he wants to watch is *Spiderman*, and I don't like it."

"Haven't you blocked Retro-TV?" I asked Chris.

"You didn't tell me to block it," he said.

"Well, it has commercials ranging from pregnancy tests to the Slap Chop. Will has them all memorized."

"Really?" Chris asked.

"Fettuccine, linguini, bikini," I said. "And First Response. 'The only test that tells you six days sooner.'"

"I'm on it," Chris said. "It's easier than parenting."

"Mom." Vivian reminded us of her presence. "I want to watch my TV shows."

I'd like to say my kids were coming down from a sugar high, but this behavior was pretty normal for us.

"William!" I screamed. "Get down here. Now."

He came.

"You need to share the TV or no one's going to watch it. No more tonight. Tomorrow, Vivian gets to choose. Now it's bedtime."

"But Mom—" Vivian began to protest.

"Bed. Now."

One hour later, I emerged downstairs, sweating from the early summer that seemed to have surrounded us. I grabbed some water since we had no beer.

"Mom?" Four feet padded down the stairs.

"For crying out loud—"

"Get back to bed," Chris said. "Your mother's exhausted."

Somehow we'd channeled our parents and the phrases they used on us thirty years before.

"Mom, I can't sleep," Will said.

"Me neither," Vivian echoed. "It's still light out."

"Yes, it is. It's called summer in Canada," I said. "And leave your blackout blinds alone."

"But kids are playing outside," Will said. "Can we play outside?"

"No," said Chris. "Their parents don't love them."

Vivian and William looked at each other, communicating something in their inaudible twin language.

"Can we play outside?"

I sighed. "No. It's way past your bedtime. It's a school night. Go. To. Bed."

"But it's hot. It's so hot I can't sleep," Vivian said.

"Well, your ceiling fan is on. If I crank it any faster, our house may end up in Kansas. I suspect it's hot there too."

"It's so hot we can't sleep," Will said.

They had a point. This was record setting end-of-May heat and second story bedrooms in a house lacking air-conditioning didn't help.

"Take off your pajamas," Chris said.

Vivian and William looked at their pjs, then to me, then back to their pjs, then to each other.

"Really?" one of them said.

I nodded.

"Can we sleep naked?" William asked.

"No. In your underwear." Visions of William sneaking his Thomas the Tank Engine up to his room crossed my mind.

They grinned. You could see the lack of privilege in my children's lives when they got excited about being able to shed their clothing.

I returned to my previously scheduled activity, wasting time on Twitter when I should have been tidying the living room.

"Mom, we're still hot," one of them said. Sometimes it was hard to keep track of which twin spoke because they talked in collective pronouns.

"Stop talking," I said. "It makes you hot."

Chris smiled.

They trundled off to bed.

Another minute, another mindless tweet.

"Mom, it's hot." William wandered down the well trodden stairs.

"Yes. It's summer. It gets hot."

"I can't sleep. I'm so hot."

This time, Chris spoke first. "If you're that hot, go stick your head in the toilet."

"Really?"

"Good night."

Although we didn't hear a flush, we also didn't hear any more noise from their bedroom. I shut my laptop. One hundred and forty characters were getting to be too much for me.

I scooted onto our living room floor and looked around me at the sea of picture books that had been thrown out of the bookcase. Chris joined my Dr. Seuss sit-in.

"Remember when we used to watch *Whose Line Is It Anyway*?" I asked.

Chris smiled. "Yes. Every Sunday night in Bangkok."

"Remember that skit where they'd put 'if you know what I mean' at the end of every sentence?"

Chris nodded. A decade together meant he knew where my mind was going.

We both grabbed a book and opened up to a random page.

I grabbed a Doreen Cronin book, opened up, and read, "*Bob had all the pigs washed in no time*, if you know what I mean."

We laughed.

"How about this one?" Chris said, picking up *The Cat in the Hat* and opening to a random page. "*And then something went BUMP! How that BUMP made us JUMP*, if you know what I mean."

We laughed until our ribs hurt.

Soon, we shortened the game. We added the double entendre phrase to the end of the titles.

"*Pat the Bunny*, if you know what I mean."

"*There's a Wocket in my Pocket*, if you know what I mean."

"*The Very Hungry Caterpillar*, if you know what I mean."

"*Where the Wild Things Are*, if you know what I mean."

But it was the final one that made me die a little death: "*Hop on Pop*, if you know what I mean."

WHO TOLD YOU THAT YOU SHOULD BREATHE THROUGH YOUR MOUTH WHEN DADDIES POO?

I'm a big fan of using choice as a way to coerce kids into doing what I want them to do.

I learned this early in my teaching career. I used to spout platitudes like, "You always have a choice, it just may not be a good choice," but I got tired of hearing teens make gagging noises. So I halted my sermonizing and started putting the philosophy into practice. When a pubescent creature was doing something highly annoying, I'd pause and offer a choice, such as "You can either stop armpit farting and stay in this classroom, or you can armpit fart all the way down to the principal's office."

This either-or strategy, a type of souped-up bribery, proved especially useful for parenting five year olds.

To Vivian, I've said: "You can either eat your carrots and have dessert, or you can leave them on your plate to fester and decay while you starve for days to come."

To William, I've said: "You can either stop sucking on that LEGO piece, or you can keep sucking on it and never watch *The Backyardigans* again, ever."

The equation of this discipline technique can be indicated by the formula: Choice + Hyperbole = Manipulation. You're solving for sanity.

I must use this technique often, because one day Vivian cornered me with her own version of Manipulation 101.

 Parenting Tip: Manipulation 101 is a highly effective discipline strategy. It is represented by the following equation: CHOICE + HYPERBOLE = MANIPULATION.

I was in the kitchen doing something useful, like boiling water for the fourth time with the hope that I'd actually remember to make a cup of tea while the water was still hot.

"Mom," Vivian said, "would you like to sit on the couch and read me a book, or would you like to sit on the floor and play Fish?"

I took a moment to process the options.

And you know what?

It worked.

A five-year-old connived me—her mediocre mother—into following her agenda.

Freaking master apprentice.

There is little choice, however, in dealing with disgusting things when you're a parent. And there are few things more disgusting than finding used Band-Aids that don't belong to you in your purse while you're eating dinner in a restaurant. The only experience that came close to out-grossing that was when I was a college student moving into an apartment. On the floor of what was to be my bedroom, my roommate and I found a goopy condom, one that was used mere hours before. I remember looking at my roommate and saying, "Well, we can rest assured that these idiots aren't procreating."

But back to the other type of sticky-bodily-fluid things: Band-Aids. No parent in their right mind goes anywhere without them.

 Parenting Tip: It is wiser to forget a child than leave your house without a Band-Aid.

The average length of time a Band-Aid stays on in our house is four minutes. I find the used ones in the bottom of the bathtub, stuck to the bottom of my sock, or plastered to the fridge door. But the greatest concentration of used Band-Aids is in my purse.

On the eve of the last day of school, Chris and I went on a date. I rifled through my purse trying to find my cell phone to check if the babysitter had called in the past ninety minutes. Chris had gone to the bathroom, and I needed to look like I was doing something. I hadn't had a chance to change purses so I was using the one that could have held a third baby if I had lacked birth control. Finally, I pulled out my cell phone. Stuck to it were two used Band-Aids. I nearly gagged, but was able to multitask effectively: drop the purse while reaching for the Shiraz.

Chris returned. "The ratio of used Band-Aids to new Band-Aids in my purse is 3:1," I told him.

He grimaced.

I held up the phone with its accessories.

"That's disgusting."

Just then our waiter came by. I hid the phone.

"Would you like another drink?" he asked.

"Would I ever," I said.

The next day, Vivian and William's last day of preschool, I should have rented a U-Haul trailer with a one-way ticket to the recycling depot. Three months later, I still hadn't sorted through folders, journals, posters, nametags, and winter newsletters that said someone in the class had lice. I hoped it wasn't one of my spawn.

Instead of doing the drop-and-dump method, I backed the minivan into the garage and made twenty-four trips into our house with crumpled construction paper. Good to know my children were glue-sticking their way to literacy.

Once I finished Operation De-Construction Paper, I made no-name Kraft Dinner; we were, after all, trying to pay back our kids' bank account. I liked to buy foods with as many unrecognizable ingredients as possible on the box as it gave William and Vivian something to read when they were waiting for dinner.

Parenting Tip: Look for opportunities to practice your child's literacy skills. Buying food with unrecognizable ingredients aids this educational pursuit.

I served dinner, if you could call it that. The food group "Beige" was well represented.

"So, what happened on your last day of school?" I asked.

"Nothing," William said.

"Right," I said. "Same as all the other one hundred eighty days?"

He kept chewing.

"I know something that happened," Vivian muttered through partially chewed macaroni. "I learned something."

"You learned something at school today? Really?" I asked. I hadn't been concerned with my sarcastic tone since I broke that New Year's Resolution on January 2.

"I learned that when daddies poo, you should breathe through your mouth."

"Really?"

"Yeah."

"Wow, the curriculum is getting more practical," Chris said.

"What does that mean, Mommy?"

"Oh, nothing."

"Who told you that you should breathe through your mouth when daddies poo?" I asked.

"A boy in my class."

"What do you think of his advice?" I asked.

"I like it."

"Me too."

"Mom," said William, oblivious to the conversation that happened, "can I have some more?"

Help yourself. Later, we'd all be breathing through our mouths.

THE SAPPY FILES, PART 4 (OR WHY MY KIDS' FUTURE THERAPISTS SHOULD BELIEVE I DON'T NEED TO BE COMMITTED. YET.)

Dear Vivian and William,

There is nothing that makes me more thankful for you both than a trip to the hospital. Adjacent to the bright LEGO-style building that is the Alberta Children's Hospital, there is a parking garage that sells monthly passes. Whenever I grab the ticket from the entrance, a multitude of emotions runs over me, from sadness for the families who've spent countless nights there, to relief that it's not us.

We were there for day surgery. For you, William. I am grateful that your dad and I didn't have to have the argument that I imagine so many other parents have had, wondering if they should purchase a weekly or a monthly pass.

We took the elevator up to the third floor to the day surgery waiting room, a kid-friendly place with bold art, toys, and cartoons on TV.

William, I remember helping you into a primary-colored hospital gown that hung down to your knees. You leaned over the train table, nearly revealing your bare butt. I pulled out puppets so your sister could entertain us. My eyes took in everything: a mother on a cell phone, a surgeon briefing a family, your absorption in the moment of play.

While waiting diaper-less, another child—a toddler girl—peed herself. The receptionist smiled, grabbed a mop, and reassured the girl's parents. "It happens all the time," she said.

There are angels everywhere.

You both seemed to sense this shift in mood and came back to your dad and me and climbed onto our laps.

How do you prepare a child for anesthetic? I wondered silently.

But William, you interrupted my thoughts. "Mom," you said, "will there be a woman and an alligator purse?"

I tried to figure out what you were talking about. Did that mom over there have a fancy purse? What movies had you watched recently?" I turned to your dad for some clarification, but he was as lost as me.

"Will," I said, "I don't know—"

"Mom," Vivian interrupted, "it's the book, *The Lady with the Alligator Purse.*"

I smiled, both at the thought of that story and at how you and your sister often understand each other immediately.

I remembered the book. In it, a boy is sick. A doctor comes in and prescribes penicillin, then a nurse suggests castor oil, but it is the lady with the alligator purse who brings the real healing power: pizza.

"I'm not sure she'll be there," I said.

Sadness clouded your face.

"We'll find her," your dad added.

Soon your name was called.

The four of us held hands and walked down a long hallway, through secured double doors, and into a wide holding area, a waiting place. Under bright fluorescent lights, your dad and I stood, every bit as unsure as we were the moment before you were born. Only this time, you and your sister held our hands. You both gave us strength.

I looked around. The only other people were a Hutterite woman and her teenage son. We exchanged smiles.

Then, a nurse and an anesthesiologist come out of the operating room and invited you to go with them.

"Maybe that's the Lady with the Alligator Purse," your sister told you.

I tried not to cling to you. I tried, but failed. Then I watched as you walked away, a pint-sized boy flanked by two medical personnel in scrubs. You walked without looking back through the swinging surgical doors.

I tried to compose myself, for your sister. I tried hard. The Hutterite woman smiled at me. In a Low German accent, she asked, "What's he in for?"

I explained. I wiped my eyes. "It's not that serious," I added. "The doctor says it's routine. Well, routine for the doctor, I guess."

"Doesn't matter," she said. "He's your boy."

Tears came. Yes, he's my boy, I thought. He may be the little s*** who first licked the minivan, the one who peed on Minnie Mouse, and the one who clobbered his sister after she was a little s*** to him, but he is my boy.

We walked back to the busy waiting room. Vivian, you walked between your dad and me, shoring each of us up with your hands.

"What do you think about ordering pizza for dinner when we all go home?" your dad asked.

Vivian, you squealed your assent and let go of our hands.

"Perfect," I answered.

And when those long hospital hours were over and we got to take both of you home, we did order pizza, just after we recycled our daily parking pass.

Good Lord, I love you both.

Always,

Mommy

PART FIVE

KINDERGARTEN, OR WHY I HAD
A BREAKDOWN

I PUT THE MENTAL IN ENVIRONMENTAL

The good thing about being a teacher is that you have the summers off with your children. The bad thing about being a teacher is that you have the summers off with your children.

In my early, delusional years of parenting, I wanted my children to grow up to be outdoorsy and to become self-sufficient, unconcerned with appearances, and able to pee in the bush. In pursuit of these three objectives, we scavenged some gear, loaded our van Joad-style, and set off for the Wild West. We left our second-hand reference book, *Camping for Dummies*, at home, where it served as a paperweight for Vivy's preschool art collection.

We were wedged into the minivan, a veritable family puzzle of gear, food, and stuff. I couldn't even see Vivy or Will. Three hours later, with the lyrics from a SpongeBob SquarePants DVD carved into my long-term memory, we descended into a valley once inhabited by dinosaurs. The fact that we were going to an area where bigger-than-RV creatures became extinct should have been my first clue that this wasn't going to be a warm and fuzzy, immortalize-it-in-a-pretty-scrapbook trip. The second omen came when the park ranger told us there'd been three rattlesnake bites in the campground that month. Stay out of long grass, he advised. And with that cautioning, I eliminated the third objective of the trip: teaching my kids to pee in the bush.

We pulled our loser cruiser into Lot 33 and began to unpack.

"That's the age Jesus was when he died," I said.

"What are you talking about?" Chris asked.

"Our lot number, thirty-three. Don't you think it has some sort of sacrificial quality to it? I turned thirty-five after you knocked me up. Being pregnant was a sacrifice."

Chris threw a box of junk food out of the van, missing my toe by an inch.

"I'll take Sunday School Trivia for $400, Alex," he added, fixated on my Jesus comment.

"Ha, ha. Very fun—" I began, until a gust of wind swept away my response, one of our unsecured tarps, and a kid.

Chris rescued the wayward tarp. "Let's set up the tent before we're blown to Montana."

Now, in most families I know, especially my own, an invitation to set up a tent marked a shift from happy-enough gathering to family fight. Setting up a campsite gives way to divorce court arguments over important matters: where the tent should go; how to hammer in a plastic peg without breaking it; whether the tent is squared or on level ground; and how concerned to be about the location of children.

Parenting Tip: Camping is the fast track to divorce court. Stay in a hotel instead, preferably without your kids. Or anyone else's kids.

"Where are the kids?" I asked, trying to jam tent poles together without breaking my blood blisters.

"Beats me."

"Have you seen the other poles?" I asked.

And then I noticed a blur of action. Will and Vivy were using two tent poles as scythes to smash through long grass. They couldn't piss off rattlesnakes more if they tried.

"Get over here, right now. The snakes are getting ready to bite you."

Lesson #1: Camping could kill you.

We continued setting up our Taj Mahal, purchased at a garage sale. We squabbled over which way the fly went, repositioned it repeatedly, always managing to get it wrong. I was about to issue a parental advisory for foul language when Chris spoke: "William. Put that #$%*ing axe down."

"You left the axe out?" I asked. "They could kill—"

"Where the heck am I supposed to put it? In the garage?"

Lesson #2: Camping could kill you.

With the axe safely lodged into a tree, we grunted the fly into place. Another gust of wind tested our plastic tent pegs, at least the ones that weren't broken. Our tent was miraculously erect, but we had little time to admire it. We were distracted by the gaggle of kids across the road, some sort of extended-cousin-mix party, where offspring out-numbered parents 13:1. They careened down the road on bikes, without helmets, practicing wipe out techniques and comparing lesions. The moms and dads were modern day versions of SCTV's Bob and Doug McKenzie: six adults drinking beer and belching around a fire.

We met our still-drunk neighbors again that afternoon on the small beach and watched neglect-in-progress as their progeny committed numerous transgressions: throwing beer bottles into the water, tossing shovels full of sand on us, and trying to provoke my son into a water fight. When one little cretin two-hand pushed Vivy into the hole she dug, we voted with our feet and left.

Lesson #3: Camping could kill you.

While roasting wieners and marshmallows over open flames for dinner, Vivy and Will found new reasons why families like ours should have the campground ambulance on speed dial: They attempted to poke each other with marshmallow forks in some sort of medieval fencing prac-tice, as they stumbled around the campfire.

Lesson #4: Camping could kill you.

Night approached. We crawled deep into our sleeping bags and awaited the beauty of nighttime silence. Instead, we were greeted by car doors slamming, the park ranger driv-ing around in his diesel truck, the neighbors arguing about who could flick their beer cap the farthest, and a generator reverberating off cliffs. Yes, the guy five sites up had powered up his generator because he was afraid the dead bodies in his freezer would go bad. Although his motor partially muted the amateur guitarist who sang "Dust in the Wind" for sixty straight minutes, the generator still sounded like a rescue helicopter circling overhead.

Lesson #5: Camping could make you want to kill.

The kids settled into a fitful sleep, and I suffered mental anguish known as The Bathroom Dilemma: Was I tired enough to fall asleep immediately, or should I crawl outside my mummy bag, trudge into darkness, and pee so that I might be able to ward off a 4:00 AM trip to the outhouse? This quandary replayed in my brain like the annoying buzz of a nighttime mosquito.

Lesson #6: Camping could make you want to kill.

Sleep eventually won until Vivy's screams trumped the generator. She blurted out, "William, stop cheating." Evidently the pinnacle of a five-year-old's nightmares is a cross between sibling rivalry and dishonesty.

Morning came, as did rain and a cold front. We put on all of our clothes and braved the outdoors. We could see our breath. We watched convoys of vehicles exit and envied the people who'd given up.

We built a fire and cooked omelets, but lost our children.

"Where are the kids?" I asked yet again.

"In the van," Chris said. "They opened and closed the door themselves. I think they even buckled themselves in. They're reading." One look at the van confirmed this. Will and Vivy, in layers of mismatched clothing and untamed hair, exiled themselves into a familiar emblem of civilization: the minivan. Though they didn't learn to pee in the bush, they had, after all, become unconcerned with their appearances and self-sufficient—in their own way.

Lesson #7: Camping was overrated.

Someday, when Vivy and Will present this book to their therapist as Exhibit A, they will call me Rain. As in on-their-parade. In addition to not taking them camping again, I also campaigned against crafts.

To punish me for my many transgressions, God gave me a daughter who fancies herself a pint-sized Martha Stewart. If Vivy could isolate enough hydrogen atoms, she'd attempt to make the sun. She loves crafts, and every adult I've ever spited has given her crafts as gifts, from the aforementioned Perler beads to scrapbooks. To me, scrapbooking is Dante's seventh circle of Hell. To Vivy, it's halfway to heaven. This could be why religion is rarely a safe topic of conversation.

One warm summer morning, as I stood in the kitchen and read reviews of movies I'd never see, Vivy pulled out one of her how-to craft books. She had already bookmarked twelve pages, which was a dozen too many.

"Can we make the castle?" she asked. "Please?"

I took my eyes off the Colin Firth movie promo. "No."

"You didn't even look at it, Mom."

I walked over to the dining room to take a better look.

I noticed a small milk spill under Vivy's chair.

"Sweetie," I said, "you spilled some milk. Can you clean it up?"

Vivy reached her foot out and stepped on it.

"Don't use your sock to do that."

"You do it all the time."

I activated my short-term memory, which was getting shorter by the hour. "Mommy does not clean the floor with her socks all the time."

"Yes, you do," Will yelled from his perch in the living room.

"Do not."

"Do too."

 Parenting Tip: To save time and cleaning supplies, mop up kitchen spills with your feet, preferably while wearing socks.

"OK," I said, being the adult for once. "Let's look at this book." I looked at the craft page that Vivy had bookmarked. It had more ingredients than a recipe for *duck l'orange*.

"The answer is still no."

"How about this one?"

I looked at the tiara on the opposite page.

"We can't do that craft. We're anti-glitter."

"What's anti-glitter?"

"It means we don't allow glitter into our house."

"Why not?"

"Because it makes a mess and Mommy hates to vacuum."

Parenting Tip: Some issues are worth taking a stand against. Be anti-glitter.

Her face fell.

"OK, Vivy," I said, grabbing the book. "How about this one?"

"I already made the fan once," she said. Her bottom lip started to quiver. I was not good with excessive emotion that was not my own.

"I have an idea," I said, smiling. "How about we make fans out of very special paper that Mommy has hidden away?"

She looked at me like I'd revealed a clue as to the Holy Grail's whereabouts. I bounded upstairs to my closet and pulled out a package of sparkly multicolored paper, the kind that can bring the staff of Michaels to their knees. Vivy followed.

"Where did you get this, Mommy?"

"I got it a long time ago when I thought I might make my own cards to give people."

"Did you ever do that?"

"No."

"Why not?"

"Because I realized I can't cut."

"You can cut," Vivy said.

"A little. But I'd rather write."

She smiled.

"Can we make cards, Mommy? I can do the cutting, and you can do the writing."

We traipsed downstairs. I grabbed my tea from the counter, closed the review of my next husband's new movie, and sat beside Vivy and her craft encyclopedia.

We started making cards.

We continued.

And continued.

The girl had stamina that would put an NFL running back to shame.

Lunchtime rolled around. I remembered I had another child and a husband.

"I'm hungry," Will said.

I walked to the kitchen. Chris came to help. Lunchtime preparation for me consisted of staring into the fridge for ten minutes, trying to use brainwaves to cook the food. In the pattern that was our marriage, Chris rescued me.

"How are you doing, Martha Stewart?" he teased.

"Fine," I said. "They're all going to end up in the recycle bin in a month, you know."

Chris smiled. "Maybe. But admit it. You're kind of having fun, aren't you?"

"I'm laughing, all right," I said, "while I put the mental in environmental."

A HOMELESS PRINCESS AND A LION PREPARING FOR A FLOOD, EXCELLENT CHOICE OF COSTUMES

I get excited about office supply stores. I skip the scrapbooking aisle and go straight for the pens, convinced that I don't have enough. Rumor has it that my mom had to hide my school supplies from me when I was a kid because I'd wear them out.

So, when my twins were about to enter kindergarten, I was as excited as they were. I'd grown up loving school, the rules, the friends, the coloring.

Vivy and Will were excited too. They tried on their backpacks and their shoes, parading around the house.

Then the morning came. No more dress rehearsals; this was the performance. I took the required pictures on the front step, and mentally compared their guaranteed-for-life backpacks with the brown leatherette briefcase I had had. We loaded Will and Vivy into the loser cruiser and began the journey. When we arrived at the school, we could feel the apprehension. Will and Vivy walked ahead, tentative steps and glances back at us, holding hands.

We followed.

I was a cliché: a photo-taking, tissue-wiping, hand-waving mom.

We deposited them with their teachers. I went to work, greeting my own students, who at age fourteen were less excited than my five-year-old offspring.

Later that evening, we talked about our first days. Vivy had experienced lots. Will not so much.

As they cleared the table, I asked them what kind of juice they wanted for their lunch tomorrow.

"You mean I have to go to school tomorrow?" Will asked.

"Yes, you have to go to school tomorrow," I said. "Did you think it was a one-time thing, like a birthday party?"

He nodded.

"Better get used to it, Will," Chris said. "You have to go to school for the next twenty years."

Full day kindergarten proved more challenging than I remembered. Back in the '70s, I remembered naptime, block-time, and recess-time. Vivy and Will's school seemed to want to teach them things, concepts I didn't learn in kin-dergarten or in the next three decades of my life. Things like dinosaurs and Van Gogh and lice.

After the planet debacle of preschool, we survived the dinosaur unit intact, with only a few bruises and one shattered ego—mine. Will and Vivy started coming home with dinosaur facts. If there was one thing I knew less about than the solar system, it was dinosaurs. I had enough trouble keeping track of yesterday's history, let alone something that happened before Fred Flintstone walked the streets of Bedrock.

I knew Brontosauruses existed and gave North America burgers big enough to tip a car and piss off Wilma, but other than that I knew only three dino details, all from *Jurassic Park*: Velociraptors were small but fast, T. rexes could crush you, and you want to be driving a luxury SUV if ever chased by a dinosaur.

Will and Vivy attempted to correct my ineptitude.

"These aren't Brontosaurus burgers," Will told me at dinner. "They're dead cow."

"Well," I said, "dinosaurs are dead, so that makes them kind of the same."

"Dinosaurs aren't just dead, Mom," Vivy explained. "They're stinked."

"I bet they're stinked," Chris said. "Sometimes Mommy's stinked too."

I rolled my eyes, a skill Vivy was starting to mimic.

"Mommy's not stinked, Dad," Will said. "She's right there."

I put some mustard on my dead cow. "What did you do at recess today?" I asked, anxious to change the subject.

"I played paleontologist," Vivy said.

I coughed. "That sounds like a disease," I said.

"Mom," Will said. "It's people who find and learn about dinosaurs.

Parenting Tip: Accept that all dinosaur names sound like diseases. Then bookmark the Wikipedia page on dinosaurs so your children don't think you're abnormally stupid.

Chris passed me the cheese. "Did you play paleontologist, Will?" he asked.

"No," he said. "I played roll-down-the-hill."

"How do you play that?" I asked.

"You roll down the hill."

I pursued an earlier conversation track.

"Vivy, you actually pretended you were a paleontologist at recess?"

"Yes."

"You didn't want to roll down the hill?"

"No. I pretended I found the bones and horns of a Triceratops."

I rolled my eyes again. Chris caught this and smiled at me. "So, when you were in kindergarten, you never pretended you were a paleontologist?"

I shook my head. "I just learned that word last year on *Jeopardy*."

"What did you play at recess, Mommy?" Vivy asked me.

"Girls-catch-the-boys," I said.

"Mommy was very good at that," Chris said.

"Still am, you mean."

If the beginning of kindergarten wasn't enough to fast track me to the liquor store, Halloween was, as the previous year had taught me. I used to love Halloween. I have fond memories of Halloween as a child filling a pillowcase of candy, and as a college student fending off drunken animals, literally. Then I became a parent, and Halloween morphed into a day that combined my hatred of crafts with bad chocolate that I ate anyway.

On the eve of Halloween, Vivy and Will hadn't yet chosen what costume they wanted to wear because, like last year, we hadn't asked. When you're five, choice is over overrated. When you're forty, choice is temptation.

"Go look in the dress-up trunk," I said. "Find a costume for tomorrow." Chris had spent twenty-nine hours and four tanks of gas collecting costumes from garage sales.

Evidently all that kindergarten talk about Brontosaurus burgers and Jupiter's gases had caused Will to grow. Because when he emerged from the crypt, he was dressed as a lion with human legs. The cute fluffy paws, meant to cover his shoes, were mid-shin. It looked even better with gym socks extending past his ankles, leaving a three-inch gap of skin. Vivy, on the other hand, was a princess of sorts. She had put on two Velcro-backed fairytale dresses, both with holes in them, leaving her with a layered look. Add to this mixture her straight hair, which formed dreadlocks minutes after combing, and we had a politically incorrect homeless princess in our presence.

Thankfully, in our community, no one started trick-or-treating until the sun set. This meant it was harder for people to see how pathetic our kids' costumes were. Last year, it was a tutu over snow pants. And that was my costume.

"Here we go," I said to Chris. "A homeless princess and a lion preparing for a flood. Excellent choice of costumes."

"You may wish to sheath your sarcasm sword," Chris added, kissing my cheek. "It may scare some kids."

"I'm good with that," I said, leaving my husband to hand out candy dressed in what he called his "cranky, middle-aged man" costume.

HER PUKE RUINED THE NEW CAR SMELL

Will and Vivy desperately wanted a pet. They would have loved a cat, but Chris is allergic to any fluff ball that meows. So our twins colluded and settled on getting a dog. I tried to avoid this debate about pets, because the odds were pretty even. When Chris was home, it was two against two; when he was out, we might have had quorum, but the dynamic duo of Vivy and Will had a definite majority.

I didn't want a dog because I didn't want more work. I'd already taught two kids not to pee on the floor: been there, done that. I was still working on the don't-lick-your-plate thing, especially on the rare evenings when we had company. In an attempt to silence the pet issue, I employed the Distant Future Strategy; in other words, I told Will and Vivy they couldn't get a dog until they were ten years old. I was banking on them forgetting about it over the next five years. That was unlikely, though, given that I first informed them about this arbitrary rule the previous year, and they still remembered. About every second day, one of them said, "I wish we were ten, Mom . . ."

They'd taken the dog-theme to heart. Not only did they bark and play fetch with each other, but on one occasion I caught Will the Puppy licking his sister's leg. Apparently, I needed to expand the don't-lick-your-plate rule to include people. After being licked on the leg, Vivy patted Will's head and said, "Nice doggie."

> Parenting Tip: Avoid getting a pet at all costs. If you do, see a psychologist who specializes in masochistic behavior psychosis.

In their relentless pursuit of getting a dog, Vivy and Will adopted a clever marketing tactic: If you can't close the big sale, go for a bunch of smaller ones.

They harped on and on about fish and hamsters. Chris compromised. "I'll give you half a hamster. If you keep it alive, I'll give you the other half."

The kids looked at him, horror-stricken.

"How would we get half a hamster?" Will asked.

"Carefully," Chris said.

"Dad, we can't keep half a hamster alive," Vivy said, "it'd be dead."

"You're right."

Later that day, I sat in my neighbor's dining room performing yet another community service: neither she nor her husband drank red wine, so when they had some I drank it for them. We talked about pets. They had definite plans to get a dog; I had definite plans to have a second glass of wine.

When they asked about my no-pet policy, I explained that it wasn't because I was anti-dog. I loved my childhood mutts; it was just that they were farm dogs, which meant that they didn't step a paw in the house, we didn't have to walk them, and we didn't own a leash. Essentially the dogs took care of themselves and once a week I'd pet them or chase them around the community trying to find out which b*tch they knocked up.

As I babbled about all this to my neighbor, she poured me a second glass. "Have you taken the kids to the pet store?" she asked. "You know, to play with the animals."

I took a sip of my wine. "They have animals there?" I asked.

She paused, taking her time to refill her own glass with Sauvignon Blanc. "What did you think they sold?"

I could tell she was reining in the sarcasm.

"Dog food? Leashes?"

On Sunday, I drove Will and Vivy to the pet store, which was five minutes away.

I confirmed that pet stores did indeed have live animals. The kids and I watched a bird squawk, petted a puppy that resembled a Muppet, and explored the aquarium section.

"Please can we get a fish?" Will asked.

"No."

"Why not?" Vivy said.

"Look, I told you this a bazillion times before. I can't even keep a plant alive."

"We'll take care of it."

And then I saw it. The writing on the wall. Literally.

It read: Thirty Day Fish Guarantee. In order for the guarantee to be valid, please ensure that you have the following with you: your original sales receipt, the body of the dead fish, separate ½ cup of water from your fish tank. Please Note: The water sample must be separate from the fish body.

I laughed. The image of being denied a refund because I had returned the dead fish body *in* half a cup of fishbowl water was vivid. And plausible.

"Let's go," I said.

And out we skipped, empty-handed.

Although pretending to be dogs and keeping decapitated rodents alive might be the talents of some members of my family, they are not mine.

When I was six, my sister dragged out a tape player the size of a poodle and recorded me hosting a *Gong Show*–style program. After all, we were farm kids with little to do in the winter. In my own kid version of *The Gong Show*, I assigned talents to my family members and rated them. My dad's skill was hammering and he pounded his way to a score of seven out of ten. My brother's talent was "blowing stinks" (also known as farting); he got gonged, as in big time, wind-up, hit-the-gong-as-hard-as-you-can gonged. Not sure what my sister's skill was, but it was no doubt pretty good. My mom's special talent was curling, as in the sport, not her hair (that was what perms were for), and she received a ten. And there you have it, my worldview at age six.

Every year, tens of people honor Celebrate Your Unique Talent Day on November 24. I asked my twins to share what they believed were the unique talents of each of us. According to Vivy, her talent was drawing cats and flowers, Will was good at silly dancing, and Mommy excelled at loving and cuddling. Daddy, according to Vivy, was good at watching basketball on TV. And she was right: He was good at that as well as at rescuing my attempts to cook.

Will then weighed in on the debate. He declared that he was good at playing computer games, which was true since he was closing in on Gladwell's 10,000-hour rule. Vivy, he claimed, was great at playing blocks. He confirmed that watching TV was Daddy's specialty. As for me? Will said my talent was sitting. Not standing, not sleeping . . . but sitting.

Somehow we survived the next month. Instead of getting a pet, we opted to spend Christmas with my parents in an RV. It seemed like a good idea at the time, since it was an easy flight to Arizona. Now, before I go any further, I'd like to nominate "an easy flight" as the stupidest term there is. If you have ever flown on a plane with young children (or been on a flight with young children), you know that "an easy flight" is, at best, paradoxical.

Parenting Tip: If you search "Advice for Traveling with Children," the number one rule is "DON'T."

So, we were on this easy flight, and it was going smoothly. Chris napped in front of a movie. Will was in paradise because when the plane took off, he was able to see what he thought was a combination of LEGOLAND and Hot Wheels from his window. When clouds obstructed his view, he was able to watch cartoons two inches from his face.

Vivy, who sat beside me, ignored the TV. In six minutes, she finished her two-week activity package that took me three hours to assemble. She was bored, but not for long. Somewhere over Salt Lake City, a puke-show started in the seat behind her. An eight-year-old girl vomited all over herself, the backs of our seats, and her mom. She continued heaving every ten minutes into a growing collection of barf bags. I gave the mother a sympathetic smile that oozed schadenfreude: I'd been there, but I was giddy that it was her this time.

Vivy, despite my protests, kneeled on her seat and peered over her headrest so she had an unspoiled view of the throw up fest. When I insisted she wear her seatbelt—a concern for confinement as much as safety—she reclined her seat, sat on one butt cheek, and craned her head so she could peer between the gap. It entertained her until we landed.

We picked up the rental car, which was the cleanest car we'd ever sat in. I pulled out my folder of Google maps that was the size of Shakespeare's complete works, and Chris started driving. Before long, we were on the interstate heading to Yuma. We cruised along, stopping only to buy some fine Mexican cuisine at a gas station.

The drive was going well, too well. And then I heard those infamous five words.

"I'm going to be sick."

"No. Don't. Wait. Hold on," I pleaded as I looked for a receptacle, anything. I emptied out a shopping bag, turned around, and kneeled on my seat, twisting my seat belt into a noose.

Too late.

Puke was everywhere: on Vivy's clothes, in her hair, on the plush seats. Upgrading to get the leather interior would have been prescient, I thought. My momentary regret was interrupted by Vivy sobbing and Will screaming, "Gross!" I joined the noisy fray and yelled at Chris to pull over.

"There's nowhere," he shouted over the chaos.

"Anywhere. An off-ramp. A freaking cactus."

Many sticky minutes later, he found an off-ramp. We got out, Chris grabbed some clothes from a suitcase, and I undressed our gooey daughter. I momentarily smirked because I'd brought a roll of paper towels; never before had I been this prepared for cleaning puke off a naked five-year-old on an Arizona interstate.

Chris threw Vivy's soiled clothes on a cactus. "We're not taking those with us." I knew this tone; it was the nonnegotiable one.

I grabbed more paper towels and started to clean the car seats. "Her puke ruined the new car smell," I announced. When I finished collecting chunks of regurgitated soft tacos, I gave Vivy a hug and a plastic bag.

"Don't stick your head all the way in it," I cautioned.

 Parenting Tip: Never travel without a Vomit Survival Kit. Ensure it includes Xanax.

DID YOU ACTUALLY LICK THE TIRE?

I wiped my hands on my pants, climbed back into the rental car, and took attendance.

"Will?" I asked. I craned my neck in the direction of the vomit smell and saw an empty booster seat. "Where's Will?"

Chris looked in the backseat, questioning my ability to conduct a search and rescue operation in a sedan.

"He's not in here," Chris said.

I comforted Vivy, who was not upset about her MIA brother as much as she was her soggy stuffed dog. Holding her hand did little to console her.

Chris exited the vehicle to expand his search field.

Through the car window, I heard him address Will in loud muffled tones. I made out the words "disgusting" and "germs," two terms that cover 95 percent of childrearing topics.

I let go of Vivy's hand.

"What happened?" I asked as testosterone reentered the vomit sphere.

"Will was licking the tire," Chris said, reaching for the collection of antibacterial products he'd already unpacked in the glove compartment.

I twisted my neck to look at Will, who was struggling with the seatbelt.

"Did you actually lick the tire?"

"Yes," he said. He had not yet learned the art of lying, blaming his sister, or farting to draw attention away from the real issue at hand.

"Why?" It was my favorite question to ask rhetorically, in a half-prayer, half-swear manner.

"I don't know."

"Did you pee on it, too?" Chris asked.

"No."

I heard the seatbelt click.

"Let's go before we have to deal with another bodily fluid," I said.

Chris put the car in gear and merged back onto the interstate.

We arrived at the RV park none too soon. Vivy's stomach was churning, Will was bored with my count-the-cacti game, and Chris was tired of driving with his head stuck out the window to avoid the smell of puke.

We stopped at the security gate. A septuagenarian with a clipboard limped to Chris's window. I was pretty sure we'd just arrived at Springfield's Nuclear Plant and were being greeted by Mr. Burns himself. Homer was nowhere to be seen.

"Where are ye headed?" he asked.

We handled this question like we handled every customs line up and security checkpoint since we'd started dating a decade ago. Chris stayed silent; I talked.

"We're visiting my parents," I said.

Mr. Burns raised his eyebrows. I volunteered more information, too much as was my habit. I told him the names of my parents, where they were from, how we were not staying with them but my mom's cousin who'd gone back to Canada for Christmas. I offered to sketch our family tree on his clipboard, but retches from the back seat distracted me. It was Will, who was either imitating his sister or coughing up a fur ball from licking the upholstered seats. Vivy slept.

Mr. Burns unleashed his weapon from a holster. He was packing a walkie-talkie.

He peppered us with more questions than we had at passport control.

Finally, he let us through with instructions to return to the office the next morning and fill out some IRS-looking forms in triplicate.

Mom and Dad's pre-lit palm tree leaned against their RV. We had arrived. We unloaded and I asked for the three things college students request after a night out: a bathroom, a bucket, and a beer.

Mom grabbed a pail and then cradled a gray-looking Vivy in a lawn chair.

Dad handed me a beer.

"I'm hungry," Will whined.

"I bought cheese sticks and yogurt," said Mom. "They're in the fridge."

I walked into their movie star RV, used some of my burglary skills to open the locked fridge, and brought Will a snack he'd eventually vomit up.

I sat down next to my dad, tossed Chris a Coke, and took the first sip of the beer I'd been cradling for the past five minutes.

We recounted the vomit fest and the negotiations that took place at the front gate. Vivy stirred, groaned, bolted upright. While still talking, I grabbed the pail and caught her puke.

I was on my way to dump the pail when I saw Will once again exploring his environment with his senses, something encouraged by his kindergarten class.

"Will you stop licking yogurt off your glasses?" I asked.

Somehow, we survived the Arizona puke-a-thon. We were all healthy for the flight home, but as good guests do, we left a gift for our hosts. My enduring memory of saying goodbye to my parents in their RV was of my mom hugging me as my dad speed-walked to the bathroom, leaned over the mini-toilet, and hurled his breakfast into the sewer. We shared everything.

Hours later, after enjoying a puke-free flight, we arrived home. The week progressed, and the few cardboard dinners

I prepared reminded my family that it was a blessing that Chris cooked most of the time. It wasn't long, though, until we had another food escapade.

When healthy, Vivy—a.k.a. Princess Squirm-a-Lot—was incapable of remaining still for anything as mundane as a meal. She didn't sit on her dining room chair as much as use it as a pommel horse, a move she'd perfected in utero. On the chair, she squatted, stood, pivoted in a series of practiced moves, plopping down onto her chair for a rest.

"Tie yourself to the chair, Princess Squirm-a-Lot," I said, as Chris doled out our favorite meal: mystery-meat-on-a-stick fresh from the barbecue. Chris is one of those men who enjoy barbecuing in all weather. The snowier, the better.

Vivian ignored my request. Soon, she wriggled from side to side and front to back over the surface of the chair like she was a gymnast whose score depended upon covering all four corners of the mat. And like the best gymnasts, she sometimes stumbled out of bounds. She was in the midst of informing us which of her kindergarten classmates had been naughty. Dishing out the dirt on other five year olds was a practice we encouraged as it reminded us that other people's children misbehaved too.

"If Toby pushes one more student," she said, "the teacher's going—"

Parenting Tip: Encouraging your children to gossip about their classmates will make you feel better about your own parenting skills.

And poof, she was gone. She'd fallen out of bounds, off the chair. Picture the scene from Looney Tunes where Wile E. Coyote sends an anvil hurtling off the cliff heading for the Road Runner, and you have a sense of the speed at which she fell. The sound of skull meeting ceramic tile gave way to a pregnant moment of silence; then a scream was born.

On cue, Will was off, a sprinter out of the blocks. Before she could crawl back onto the chair and reach for another cube of meat, he presented a stuffed animal. "Don't worry, Vivy," he said. "I fall off chairs all the time." It was a lie, the kind I liked. Maybe there was hope, at least for the children.

DO YOU WANT TO COME TO STRIPPER BARBIE'S FUNERAL?

January marched on like a polar bear stalking its prey. The snow kept falling; Chris kept barbecuing. By the last week, I'd had it, frustrated with temperatures that required I plug in my van, that froze my eyelashes together, and that stuck kids' tongues to bus windows.

Feeling cabin bound, I took the kids to an office supply store to get a wireless router. Maybe, I thought, I'd feel less captive in my house if I could roam freely with my laptop, not held hostage by a cord in Chris's office, surrounded by his tacky collections. If the cold didn't do me in, then the fake gorilla skull, Communist propaganda, or can of alligator meat might.

"Be good," I said, as I whisked Will and Vivy inside the red automatic doors of stationery heaven. I wandered over to the computer section with my kids in tow.

"Can I help you?" a sixteen-year-old pimpled cutie asked me.

He could. He explained what kind of router I needed, the cost effectiveness of different brands, and how to use simple technology to take down a spy satellite.

Vivy and Will danced and giggled, seemingly playing hide and seek amid the mid-aisle displays. I caught them looking at me and bursting into laughter, but that was nothing new.

Eventually, I pulled a Homer Simpson and selected the second cheapest router. I took it, paid, and marched us into the Arctic air.

Halfway to the car, I saw a mitten-less Will fiddling with his jacket pocket. "What's in there?" I asked. "Your mitts?"

"No, I left them in the car."

I stopped, faced Will, and repeated, "What's in there?" I could see my breath hang in the air, accompanying his guilt. He looked at Vivy, who shook her head at him.

He pulled out a pen—a squat pen with a face and funky plastic hair.

"William," I said. "You can't take a pen. That's stealing. We're going back to the store."

He looked down and fiddled with his back pocket. He pulled out two more pens.

"William? How many more do you have?"

We stopped in the entry and did an inventory. Then we walked to the cashier and put them on the counter.

"Tell the woman you're sorry you stole seven pens," I said.

"Sorry," Will said.

The teen girl—who I half suspected had a crush on tech boy—smiled and took the pens back.

As we walked out into the frozen tundra, I continued my lecture, saying words like "police," "jail," and "no TV."

I unlocked the van and we entered in silence.

I looked back to see if Vivy and Will had fastened their seat belts. What my eyes fell on, however, were Vivy's hands, in particular the funky pen in one.

"Where did you get that pen?" I said. Pointing-out-the-obvious was one of my few parenting strategies.

"Staples."

"You didn't think you should have told me when Will returned the seven of his?"

"Sorry."

"Out. Both of you. Back to Staples. Now."

"Mom?" said Vivy, as I opened the van's side door.

"Yes?"

"I took five pens."

"Five? Vivian!"

"Sorry. I'm really, really sorry. Mommy, I'm so sorry, I really am."

She *sorried* herself all the way to the cashier who rolled her eyes.

I drove home in silence.

"We have to call Grandma," I said. As a semi-functioning adult, I'd learned what to do when I couldn't handle things, like cooking a turkey or dealing with thieves. I tell my mom.

"Are you going to tell her we stole pens?"

"No," I said. "Today's her birthday."

"How old is she?" Vivy asked.

"Sixty-eight. No. Sixty-nine I think."

"Is she dead yet?" Will asked.

"No, Grandma's not dead yet," I said. "You just saw her in Arizona three weeks ago."

Once we established that Grandma hadn't kicked the can, winter marched on. Eventually Will and Vivy needed a bath.

Even though they rarely shared a bath anymore, they sometimes opted to. Playtime in our soaker tub was like a day at the beach, complete with beach toys, soggy towels, and high surf warnings. I played lifeguard, sitting on the toilet seat and thinking about what I'd do when my shift was over. This particular day, Vivy and Will took in the latest dollar-store toy Chris had purchased for them: Scooby Doo fake shaving cream with a blade-less razor. While they made Santa Claus beards, I became absorbed in an overdue library book, *The 4-Hour Work Week*, which could not have been written by a parent.

My focus drifted to places it shouldn't, such as dreams of four-hour workdays, life without kids, and Colin Firth.

A flying shark and giggles ruined that reverie.

"Look at us, Mom," Vivy said.

I looked. Birds' nests made from shaving cream adorned their heads. Then I looked more closely. "You're shaving each other's backs?" I asked.

They nodded and continued their barbershop act.

I sighed.

Parenting Tip: When your kids start shaving each other's backs, it's time for them to take separate baths.

"Your hair looks funny, Mom," Will said.

I felt it. The humidity of the bathroom had increased its puffiness.

"You're a fluffy puppy," Will said.

"Thanks," I mumbled. I thumbed my way to the back of the book in search of an index. "Nannies" was not in there. Neither was "boarding school."

Water hit me.

"Enough," I snapped. "Time to get out. You still need to brush your teeth. And floss too."

They looked at me.

"You're going to the dentist in four days. She's going to yell at you if you don't floss." I knew it was never too early to teach kids two important skills: cramming and using fear as a motivator.

Parenting Tip: A regular routine of brushing and flossing is essential the three days before your children's dental appointments if you want to appear to be a good parent.

Will and Vivy looked at me. I smiled, that fake smile that looks like I'm hiding severe indigestion. I knew full well that the dentist or her hygienist would ask them if they floss. I also knew that my kids wouldn't lie. I became spin-doctor Mommy.

"Can we play a bit longer?" Vivy asked.

"Sure. You can shave each other's backs for five more minutes."

Every International Women's Day, I sacrifice a slutty toy to the great landfill in the sky. Because what says "International Women's Day" like violently destroying a piece of plastic my daughter loves?

It started with the shoes. These red plastic shoes that Vivy loved to wear around the house. They were that special type of plastic, the kind that was always either too big or too small and had a grip comparable to Bambi learning to stand on ice.

I have nothing against red fancy shoes. I have a pair of peep-toe, three-inch heels that remind me I used to be sexy, I'm as tall as my husband, and I have bunions that Paul Bunyan himself would have had fun chopping off.

But Vivy's hand-me-down shoes were heeled and made from the carcinogen family of plastics. My original approach to dealing with Vivy's red shoes of death involved denial: I tossed them into the dress-up box before a trip to the ER was required. Then, a month or so later, I'd hear the clip clop of uncertain steps again.

So, when Will and Vivy were still in preschool, I destroyed the shoes. It involved a hammer, some cursing, and two Band-Aids.

With our twins now in kindergarten, it was time to up the ante. I destroyed the toy Chris nicknamed "Stripper Barbie." Stripper Barbie was a hand-me-down doll that came shirtless. Besides being topless, Stripper Barbie had a button you could press that made her hot pink skirt light up and spin. Whenever the skirt twirled, it resembled Linda Blair's famous head spin in *The Exorcist*.

In fact, seeing Stripper Barbie in action made my head spin. One week prior to Stripper Barbie's funeral, Vivy had been playing with her and four other dolls when she decided to do show and tell.

Vivy held up Stripper Barbie and said, "Isn't she beautiful, Mom?"

I ignored the question. "Which one's smart?" I asked.

Vivy held up a fully clothed doll.

"Which one's funny?"

Vivy held up another fully clothed doll.

"They're all in a movie," Vivy announced.

"They are?" I asked. I looked back at Stripper Barbie. "But where's her shirt?"

"She doesn't wear one. Not in this kind of movie," she said.

My eyes bulged, becoming bigger than Barbie's boobs.

Great, I thought. Stripper Barbie's in a porn flick.

One week later, when Will and Vivy slept, I stood at the door of our bedroom and asked Chris, "Do you want to come to Stripper Barbie's funeral?"

"Did she finally die?" he asked.

"Not really," I said. "I'm de-skankifying our house."

"You're euthanizing Stripper Barbie?"

"Yup."

"Don't you think that's a bit excessive?"

"Excessive is my style," I said. "Do you want to come to her funeral?"

"You're holding a funeral?"

"Well, I'm going to give Stripper Barbie her Last Rites as I wave her over the garbage."

"I think I'll stay here."

"OK," I said.

Chris looked up from his book. "How come you didn't have a funeral for Ken doll when the kids decapitated him?"

"I don't know."

Chris continued his questioning. "Is our family the doll mafia? Are you going all Tony Soprano on me?"

Tony? Nope. *Carmela Soprano?* Maybe.

I walked away with the doll. Minutes later, in honor of International Women's Day, Stripper Barbie went to the Great Beyond, also known as the landfill.

R.I.P., Stripper Barbie.

IF YOU CAN'T STOP LAUGHING, THINK OF SOMETHING SAD, LIKE DEAD PUPPIES

Given that Will and Vivy had thus far survived puking in Arizona, camping with rattlesnakes, and their parents, I decided to try harder to inflict pain. I took them to get their H1N1 shots to protect them from the deadly flu that never came.

True to my haphazard approach to parenting, I didn't go prepared. No snacks, no games, no distractions for the lineup. I was spinning plates to entertain two kids already hyper from chocolate cake they had consumed earlier that afternoon at a birthday party.

We began Operation Distraction by playing I Spy. I was pretty proud of Will and Vivy's progression on this game. We started playing it as a stuck-in-traffic diversion when they were two years old. I'd issue challenging clues like, "I spy . . . mommy," and both kids would point at me. Not exactly the Harvard version. Standing in that dim hospital hallway, we graduated to colors. It all went swimmingly; as we inched forward, new posters and doors offered a rain-bow of possibilities. Soon, however, the line slowed and the options dissipated. It was Will's turn. "I spy something black," he said. I followed his eyes. He was staring at the boy in line behind us, a recent immigrant from the Sudan, whose mom I'd chatted with earlier.

"All right, let's play something different. How about rhymes?" I paused. "Name one word that rhymes with car."

"Star," Vivy said.

"Bar," said Will, eyes shining, as if he knew where I'd rather be.

"Here's another one," I said. "Tell me a word that rhymes with truck." You don't need the punch line to know where this joke went. It fell in the "Mommy's not too swift" category.

We progressed to Simon Says. After I jumped up and down for half a minute, a nurse uttered that beautiful word, "Next."

We walked to Station Twelve in the final row. Vivy opted to go first. It seemed like a good idea until she saw the needle lying in wait on the table. Then she started screaming, "No, Mommy, no!" I attempted to wriggle up her sleeve, but it was too tight. Great. More clothes that didn't fit.

"You'll have to remove her shirt," the nurse said. I twisted it off and snagged Vivy's glasses in the process.

The nurse gave me precise "gripping instructions" that seemed more complicated than when Vivian was an eighteen-month-old awaiting her immunization: sit my daughter sideways on my lap, pin her right arm between my back and the chair, and hold her left arm down with my other hand. Will watched the entertainment unfold before him. Vivy caught a glimpse of the needle approaching her arm. She screamed, "I'm not ready yet!" Her enunciation and volume caused all stations to pause.

H1N1, Take Two. Vivy squirmed into a back arch that nearly catapulted her over the table, while screaming,

"I need another minute!" She's got some serious potential as a B horror film actor if her career as a one-girl-craft-factory doesn't work out.

H1N1, Take Three. She saw it coming. Her eyes were wild and she bucked like a bull-rider at the rodeo. The nurse gripped Vivy's bicep. She meant business. Vivy screamed, "Didn't you hear me? I said I need another minute!"

And the needle pierced Vivy's flesh. A shriek echoed throughout the hospital auditorium. There was a silence underneath the scream as all eleven stations once again stopped to watch the freak show. I scanned the area, making eye contact with them all. No sense pretending this wasn't my kid.

 Parenting Tip: When your child freaks out in a public space, glare at every person staring at you. Learning to "tell off" strangers with a glance is a useful skill. Practice on your spouse.

Will, transfixed by his sister's episode, was a postscript to the whole ordeal. He sat still, watched the needle prick his epidermis, and whispered, "Ouch."

When we returned home, Chris was back from work. "How did it go?" he asked

Vivy looked at her Band-Aid and said, "It was fine, Daddy."

And it was fine. Now. At least for her. I sunk into our time-out chair as deeply as I could, thoughts filled with what I couldn't articulate: birthday parties, swimming lessons, doctor's appointments, teaching, grading, filling out school forms, thank-you notes. And our kids didn't even know how to ride bikes. Not even on training wheels. That last fact crushed my heart and elevated my guilt.

Eventually, I shelved my Guilty Mother Syndrome for a while. I managed to do a useful parenting task: collect used Band-Aids on my bare feet.

I think a great gift for new parents would be stock options in Band-Aid. Let's face it: If you have a young kid, Band-Aids are an accessory. In my early days of parenting, I was anti-Band-Aids. *Tough kids don't need 'em*, I reasoned. So I made a rule: No Band-Aids unless you're bleeding.

I thought this was quite clever, and it worked well enough when Will and Vivian were two. Our consumption of Band-Aids was below average. The rule enabled us to rake in a savings of about twenty-five cents a month, not even enough to get an extra shot of chai.

My Scrimp-on-Band-Aids, Save-for-College theory— like my breasts—eventually went south. One early spring Saturday, we went to the front yard where Vivy and Will played with sidewalk chalk, which is the perfect craft for an Anti-Craft Mom since it involves no cleanup unless your kid runs onto the road and gets smushed.

Parenting Tip: If you live in a rainy climate, sidewalk chalk is the perfect craft.

So there Will and Vivy were, playing hopscotch on their crooked squares. I was flinging grape-sized gravel off our dead lawn. I looked at our Dandelion Seed Factory and shuddered. *I'm a farm girl who can't even grow grass*, I thought. And then came the screams.

I wandered over.

"Mommy," Vivy sobbed. "I need a Band-Aid."

The knee looked like classic road rash: pink and inflamed but not bleeding. "No blood, no Band-Aid," I said, hugging her.

I went back to flinging gravel pieces.

I'm not sure how much time passed until I noticed my kids were quiet.

I looked up and saw them huddled together, inspecting something.

I walked over.

Both twins were using their fingernails, scratching Vivy's scrape.

"What are you doing?" I asked.

"Nothing," they chimed, the mantra of the guilty.

"Are you picking the scrape?" I asked.

Four eyes looked up at me. Will answered, "We're trying to make it bleed."

"So I can get a Band-Aid," Vivy added.

I am losing it, I thought.

Parenting Tip: When you ask your children a question, the reply "nothing" means they're guilty. Either investigate or hide.

After the chaos of the day and dinner, we usually spent evenings in the living room. Typically, Will and Vivy took many minutes to clean up fourteen toys. Often I just did it. Then we'd play crazy, made-up games like "Cirque du Soleil: The Uncoordinated Version" and "Jump Over Mommy."

The former involved me lying on my back, bending my knees, and lifting Vivy or Will into the air and bouncing a twin on my legs. It was a good quad workout, one that I would have benefitted from doing twenty hours a day.

To play "Jump Over Mommy," I lay on the carpet and my kids two-foot hopped over me. This game helped work my abs because I would tense every time a twin leapt. It was all fun until someone landed on my face. It was Will.

He kept backing up his starting position. I had my eyes closed, but I felt it, a kick to my jaw, a shin on my nose, and a knee on my eye.

"Please don't jump on my face," I said, crawling to the couch.

"Sorry, Mom," Will said. "Can I get you a stuffy?"

I wiped my nose on my sleeve. Then I realized I was wearing a tank top. I looked from the fresh smear on my deltoid to Will. "No thanks. Just play something with Daddy. I need a time out."

Bedtime was difficult. Even though our twins were good sleepers, the evening hours sucked the life out of me. I prided myself on being the parent who tucked them in, the mom who recited a nightly blessing, the English teacher who read aloud to them using different voices for each character. But really, once you experience endless numbers of bedtimes without a break in the routine, it becomes a chore, even if it's a chore you opt for. Bedtime was a dangerous mathematical formula that had been tested time and time again: tired children + desperate parents = fast track to epic meltdown and/ or therapy. When you had twins who slept in the same bedroom, it was like your kids were having a slumber party 489 nights a year. There was jumping on beds, giggling, slamming doors, scaling closets, hiding and (sometimes) seeking, constructing forts, and chucking pillows.

> Parenting Tip: Always remember the formula for disaster: TIRED CHILDREN + DESPERATE PARENTS = EPIC MELTDOWN.

One night during that long spring, Will and Vivy would not settle. They were in that overtired, on-the-edge giggling phase, and neither repeated warnings nor empty threats would calm them down. Everything produced a giggle: their stuffed animals, their elbows, even spitting on themselves.

I'd had it.

"You need to stop laughing," I said, as the clock ticked past 9:30.

More giggles.

"Look, I'm serious," I pleaded. They didn't seem to get that, for once, I was serious. "Stop laughing and go to sleep."

More giggles.

Vivy paused for air long enough to utter, "We can't." For reasons unknown, this two-word sentence sent Will into hysterics.

"We . . . can't . . . stop . . . laughing," Vivy repeated.

"OK, if you can't stop laughing, think of something sad," I said.

"Like what?" Will challenged.

I leaned against the frame of their bedroom door. "Like dead puppies," I said.

For a moment, there was silence. Both kids looked at me with big, unblinking eyes, eyes that proclaimed bewilderment and innocence and shock. Then Will turned his head to Vivy, and they exhaled simultaneous giggles, breaking into lie-on-their-backs laughter.

I shut the door. I walked to our bedroom. I crumbled. For good this time.

The final score = Kids 2, Dead Puppies 1, Mom 0.

I CAN'T COPE ANYMORE

Pneumonia took me down in April. Insomnia, anxiety, and depression filled the void in May. And June. And part of July.

"I can't," I told Chris. "I can't cope anymore."

I couldn't believe I let this happen. Again.

Slowly, over agonizing weeks and months, I realized that I didn't have to do it all. Chris picked up and held each piece of me. I began to breathe. And sleep.

I became whole again, a different whole.
A Picasso-like whole.
And eventually, my humor returned. Halle-freaking-lujah.

THE SAPPY FILES, PART 5 (OR WHY MY DAUGHTER'S FUTURE THERAPISTS SHOULD ADORE HER)

Dear Vivian,

You are a word lover. I noticed it most this year when words and coherent thoughts left me. Searching for signs of the old me in abandoned journals, I found fragments of poetry you'd spoken.

Ever since you started to speak, you've played with words, twisted them, and created something wholly new with them. A long time ago, a famous poet named Coleridge defined poetry as "the best words in the best order." You, my love, are our poet in residence.

One day, you walked up to me in the kitchen, climbed onto the counter, and said, "Did you know human beings are made of love?"

I've saved some of my favorite lines of yours in dog-eared notebooks. It's time to give them back to you.

On a warm spring day: "Let's go watch the flowers grow."

In a park with natural landscaping: "Can we walk through the heavenly grass?"

Seeing trees covered in hoar frost: "They look like snowflakes standing up."

On saying goodbye to me for two nights: "You're a come-back-er woman."

After reading a beloved book: "A kissing hand smells like love."

Before bedtime: "When I yawn, my brain sounds like a cloud moving by."

Waiting for Grandma to arrive: "My heart is filled with bursting love."

After I left for a conference: "My heart is a little smaller when Mommy is away."

Advising me on how to swing: "Barefoot is always best."

Defining your playful father: "Adults are grown up kids."

On eating beets for the first time: "They taste like kisses covered in soil."

Carpe diem, Vivian. Thank you for teaching me to observe, to record, and to listen, and most of all, to find poetry and laughter everywhere, especially in you and your brother. Somehow, family, when it's done right, reminds me that—as broken as I've been this year and as broken as I am—I am good enough.

Much love,

Mommy

PART SIX

BEYOND KINDERGARTEN, OR PUTTING THE FUN IN DYSFUNCTION

STOP USING YOUR STRAW TO SUCK UP SPAGHETTI

We changed many things from that point on. Chris took on *all* the cooking, *all* the grocery shopping, and *all* the laundry. We hired a cleaning lady five hours per month. At Chris's insistence, I started writing every Saturday afternoon.

Will and Viv started first grade, and I registered them in Friday afternoon music lessons because I wanted my kids to learn how to do something.

I don't know what moron invented *parented* music lessons, the ones where Mom or Dad has to be present and assist. My guess is that it was some capitalist upstart who hoped to crack the Forbes 500 list before he hit thirty. It clearly wasn't a parent.

What happened to the music lessons of yesteryear, which involved dropping your kid off at the house of an elderly woman, then going alone to a smoke-filled coffee shop to pass the time? And now music lessons are *fun*. Fun? Back in the day, music students just put in time. Playing the organ, as I once did, had nothing to do with fun.

Being stupid, Chris and I enrolled Will and Viv in one of those fun, parented music lessons. After we re-mortgaged our house to pay the fees, we bought a keyboard. *Better a $100 used keyboard than a piano*, I thought. Not that we could wedge a 500-pound behemoth amid our Hoarders-R-Us style of decorating even if we wanted to.

Because we had twins, the music teacher told me that both Chris and I both would have to attend each music lesson. Now, before I go any further, it's important to mention that I'm pretty sure Chris's kindergarten report card read, "Does not play well with others." Although he would singlehandedly hold off a mob to protect his family, he is not a group man, nor does he enjoy new situations. So, when we arrived at a music studio the size of a walk-in closet, he wasn't pleased that he had to squeeze himself onto the floor between six kids, six keyboards, six women, and enough puppets to make one believe Jim Henson was still alive.

After learning a song that would be stuck in my head the rest of the year, keyboard time began. Chris flipped. It wasn't the insidious theme song that sent him over the edge, but the fact that Will played the black keys with his forehead.

"I'm taking him out to the car," he said.

"No, you're not."

A mini-domestic argument ensued, with the teacher refereeing.

After the length of time it would take to read *War and Peace* aloud in Pig Latin, the lesson ended, and all four of us left, three in silence and Viv belting out the song I wanted to forget.

The week passed slowly, and practice times more slowly still. Trying to make two six-year-olds practice after their first lesson was not that difficult; however, trying to make two six-year-olds practice what they were supposed to was—especially when they'd discovered that their electronic keyboard had a "sound effect" key. If they played middle C, they got a rooster crowing. If they played another key, an AK-47 assaulted their ears.

With the discovery of that magical button, practice time was as easy as locking kids in a pantry with freshly made cookies and asking them to refrain.

Still, onward I soldiered, insistent that my kids would practice what they were supposed to so neither would be the worst student at the next lesson.

> Parenting Tip: As long as your child isn't the worst in his class, he will succeed. If he is the worst, drink more wine.

"Will, come on," I urged. "Just play it one more time. Please?" Begrudgingly, he began.

"Mommy will be right back," I said. "Keep playing." I went to look for alcohol. As I shut the fridge door, the music changed. "William," I yelled. "Playing the vomit key does not count as practicing music."

At that point, I gave up. Whether it was the vomit key, the helicopter key, or the rooster key, the kids were practicing something.

Driving to the second lesson, I hatched a plan to prevent Chris from going ballistic. "OK," I said to him, "your job is to be Viv's dad and to pretend that Will is not your kid. So when he's crab-walking under the keyboards or using his elbows to play, I'll handle it. All you have to do is give me a sympathetic smile. Got it?"

"So I can just eye you like you're a hot mom I've never slept with?" He winked.

I smiled. Chris never got the chance, though. Minutes later, when we walked into the studio, the teacher said to him, "You know, you really don't need to be here. One parent is enough. Why don't you go have a coffee?"

Yup, Chris had managed to get himself kicked out of a parented music class. I'm pretty sure he did his happy dance when the door closed behind him. And I'm pretty sure I heard the AK-47 key go off in my head.

Sometime during that first month of music lessons, I decided that if I were going to miss happy hour with my teaching colleagues on a Friday to learn about Captain Natural and turtle-shaped half notes, then I should at least get to go out for dinner afterwards.

This epiphany came on the drive home. I didn't want to cook. I didn't want Chris to cook either since we had no groceries. I careened into our driveway, and Viv hopped out to run into the bathroom. I followed.

I should have know better than to leave Will unattended in the garage. Usually, he'd discover another Rubbermaid crate of LEGO that Chris had purchased at a garage sale, or a power tool that could render him limbless. Granted, a lack of limbs would make it harder for him to sneak out to the garage, but I preferred my son's self-mutilation to be limited to picking his cuticles until they bled.

Lying somewhere between the Dremel and the Ode-to-Star-Wars LEGO collection were the bike helmets. Chris subscribed to the theory that more was better, so why buy one full-priced bike helmet that fit your child when you could purchase twelve slightly cracked helmets that were too big or too small? It was the Goldilocks approach to outfitting children, though rare was the day that we got to the "This one's just right" resolution.

With Viv in the house already, I clambered up the garage stairs armed with purses, backpacks, lunch bags, and music bags. Once in the kitchen, I unloaded my donkey self and noticed grocery bags on the counter. Thanks to Chris, we had food again.

"Can you help me put them away?" he asked.

I grumbled the Marge Simpson back-of-the-throat growl I'd perfected, forgetting how lucky I was. I dropped my own bags and began flinging gummy bears into the pantry like they were going into forced hibernation. Viv showed me her athleticism by scaling our side-by-side freezer with frozen fish stick and bagel gear. The real challenge was to get the boxes in there and slam the door before an avalanche of insta-dinners hit you. She was good at this. She'd been in training for a while.

"Where's Will?" I asked.

Viv readjusted her grip on the freezer's top shelf. "I don't know," she said. "I think he's still outside."

I put down my comfort food—a jar of peanut butter the size of a Smart car—and headed out to the garage.

I hip-checked the door. And there he was, one six-year-old circling on his bike.

"Hi Mom," he said. "I have a helmet on."

And he did. It didn't matter that it was sitting vertical on the back of his head, not unlike how female graduates in the 1980s wore their mortar board so that it—and their hair—could defy gravity.

"Hey, Will," I said. I looked at the concrete floor and saw a collection of bike helmets strewn all over. He was using them as traffic cones. I walked over and picked them up.

And that was when I noticed it. One old pink helmet, the kind with no vent holes, lay upwards, like a bowl. And there was something in the bowl.

"Will?" I said. "Did you put water in that bike helmet?"

He smiled.

"Oh no. You didn't. Not your sister's," I stammered.

His smile widened.

"Will? Peeing in your sister's bike helmet is not a good idea."

"I know."

"It's disgusting. Why would you do that?"

"I had to pee."

"We have a toilet."

"I didn't want to take off my shoes. And you said I shouldn't pee in the front yard anymore."

"Right. Don't ever do that again," I said. "And don't tell your sister. Or your father."

I picked up the newfound potty, kicked off my shoes in the back entrance, and disposed of the entire helmet.

"Mom?" I heard from the kitchen. "Can you help me? I can't get the fries back in the freezer. And things keep hitting me on the head."

"I'll take over," I said, relieved she didn't ask to wear a helmet.

Chris took one look at me and listened to my Friday-night-dining-out proposal. He agreed, especially with the part about me needing a glass of wine.

We seemed to have more luck teaching Will and Viv about manners in restaurants.

We first started with "May I please have . . . ." Next in the series of lessons on how to appear to be more evolved than a dog came the "side order."

Viv got this immediately. "May I please have the chicken fingers with a side of salt?"

Will, too, was a quick study. "May I please have the ketchup with a side of spaghetti?"

I smiled again. There is nothing that makes a nuclear family look more Pleasantville than smiles and nods.

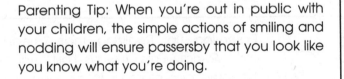

Parenting Tip: When you're out in public with your children, the simple actions of smiling and nodding will ensure passersby that you look like you know what you're doing.

Chris ordered something healthy, and I ordered last.

"What's your house red?" I asked.

Viv held up her Crayola.

I ignored her.

"I'll have the Shiraz," I said.

"Mom," Viv said. "You forgot your manners."

Right.

"May I please have a big glass of Shiraz?"

Viv's smile oozed condescension.

We colored the paper tablecloth. I drank wine. Our kids blew bubbles and saliva in their chocolate milk. I drank wine. Chris pretended to listen to me while watching the baseball game on a TV suspended over my head.

A magician who could double as a pedophile wandered over and pulled random objects out of my kids' ears while making a few bad sports jokes that involved the word "balls." I drank.

The food came.

"Say thank you," I instructed, moving my wine glass closer to me.

And we began that beautiful family time together, known as the MEAL, which stands for Mommy Eats, Always Last. For moms with young children, their own caloric consumption only happened when nearly every family member had finished.

 Parenting Tip: Realizing that "meal" stands for "Mommy Eats, Always Last" will help you become accustomed to choking down cold food.

I ate my burger, making some remark about my iron level being down because Chris insisted on eating fish four times a week in the name of health or upping our mercury levels.

I passed Viv a napkin. And another one. And one more still.

I looked over at Will, who added spaghetti to his bowl of ketchup. He was being remarkably neat, albeit inefficient.

I said, "Stop using your straw to suck up spaghetti."

"But Mom," he explained after a slurp, "I invented this. It's called a Spaghetti Sucker Upper."

"Right. Well stop using your Spaghetti Sucker Upper. Now, Edison."

"Hey," Chris said, talking to the TV, "they're calling the bullpen. You'll never guess who's going to close."

"I need more wine," I said.

My Sanity Sucker Upper was in overdrive.

YOU CAN'T SHOOT PEOPLE IN CHURCH

I don't remember learning to skate; I just remember doing it. Like most rural Canadian kids, I could walk out the back door to a natural ice surface. By the time January rolled around, however, the snow was usually too heavy to clear. Instead, we'd head to the rink on Friday night for public skating. Mom and Dad would down a few rum and Cokes while we'd play crack-the-whip and make skating trains long before the helmet era.

Will and Viv didn't have this luxury. I was not about to build a skating rink in our backyard like my outdoorsy brother did in his gentrified neighborhood. My main excuse was that we lived on a hill, but that just concealed the fact that I hated tying skate laces. It was also why I didn't do crafts or perform open-heart surgery: they all required a dexterity I did not possess.

Viv and Will took skating lessons, as in the beginner I-can't-stand-up kind. They may have held the record for being the only six-year-old Canadians who didn't know how to skate, which was rather embarrassing since both Chris and I were once proficient on blades.

Instead of sucking it up and teaching them, I took the middle-class approach, signed up my kids for skating lessons, and told Chris he was going to take them. He agreed without complaint, likely because memories of my post-pneumonia-insomnia crash remained a little too fresh in both our minds.

Parenting Tip: Paying other people to teach your children things you're more than capable of teaching them is a perfectly acceptable middle-class folly.

Ten minutes before they had to leave for the first lesson, Viv was wearing her pink ankle socks that were the thickness of tissue paper. I asked her to put on socks that were longer and thicker. She explained—rightly—that she didn't have any.

"Put on a pair of Will's," I said.

"I don't want to wear his," she said. "They're boy socks."

"No, they're not. Mommy has socks like that."

Her eyes widened, her resolve stiffened. "People will think I'm a boy."

"No, they won't."

"Yes, they will."

"No, they won't."

"Yes, they will."

"Viv, you look like a girl."

"They'll see my boy socks."

"No, they won't."

"Yes, they will."

Viv ratcheted up to full freak-out mode: screaming, tears, and tantrums.

"Vivian? Now."

"No."

"Yes."

"I'll look like a boy."

"No, you won't. You have long hair," I said, abandoning logic.

"They'll think I'm a boy."

It was at that point I said, "You don't look like a boy because you don't have a penis."

Viv responded, "No one will see that I don't have a penis."

Indeed.

And amen to that.

Parenting Tip: When you're debating with children, abandoning logic will help you win.

Will and Viv survived their first skating lesson. By the fifth lesson, I decided to go watch. Chris assured me that I wouldn't have to tie any skates, that I could bring a mug of tea into the arena, and that this was entertainment most people would pay for.

We arrived at an urban arena filled with kids attempting to stand upright on two sharp blades, trying not to be the domino that took down the row.

At the first lesson, Chris informed me, the whole class had practiced standing up. Now, I understood why they focused on that skill. Will and Viv were experts at standing up. Let's just say they'd had a lot of practice.

So, there I was on Saturday afternoon, watching eager kids gather in a circle, shifting and pseudo-listening to their teacher.

In a millisecond, one was down.

"Sniper fire," Chris said.

I looked at him for an explanation.

"One just got taken out," he said. "It looks like sniper fire."

In the time my brain took to process this, he said, "Sniper fire. Another one down." One moment Viv was standing, the next she was flat on the ice.

Sniper fire amused us for the rest of the lesson. Nothing like laughing at your own kids to make you feel better.

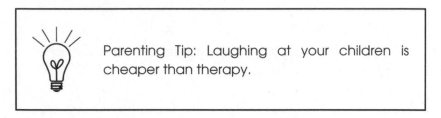

Parenting Tip: Laughing at your children is cheaper than therapy.

That autumn, not only did Viv and Will learn to stand up on skates, they also learned that Mommy likes them to go outside by themselves.

Our fenced backyard was a regulation-size chicken coop for twins. I could open the patio door, send them out, and make a cup of tea. Sometimes I looked out the window; usually I sat in silence. When I was vying for a Parent-of-the-Year nomination, I'd crack open a screen door to add an extra dimension.

One nice fall day, I sent Will and Viv outside so I could read an entire article in the newspaper, something I hadn't accomplished since the Olympics were in Athens. I think I was three-quarters through the story when I heard a shrill, trip-to-emergency scream. Three bounds later, I located the yeller. It was Viv.

I sat my butt on the grass and dragged her onto my lap. Between shrieks, I managed to hear, "William . . . croquet . . . hit . . . head."

I looked up and saw Will kicking tufts of grass. He had yet to flee the scene of the crime.

After administering basic first aid, which involved placing a Band-Aid on Viv's hair, I interrogated the suspect and the victim.

It was at that point I said these words: "Did you hit your sister on the head with a croquet mallet on purpose?"

From confessions and evidence, it appeared that Viv had taunted Will, who reacted by throwing a croquet mallet in the air. Viv's head got in the way of gravity.

No blood, no concussion, and no more croquet. But with winter on its way, the hockey sticks would soon be out. One word: duck.

The mischief of autumn led to winter, and eventually it spread beyond the fenced area of our yard and to church.

If you ever deceive yourself into believing your children are angels, take them to a small church. Or a mosque. Or any place angel-ly.

If you don't believe me, here are ten churchy things Will and Viv have done that have made me want to crawl under a pew, curl up into the fetal position, and pray that the Second Coming is imminent—like in the next thirty seconds:

1. During the sermon, Will started playing a loud version of I Spy, the colors version again. He started with "I spy something gray." It's an aging congregation.

2. When the choir started singing, Will put both hands over his ears and kept them that way for the length of a concerto.

3. When I led the children's craft class before the service, Viv asked if she could have more fairies for her cross. "They're angels," I said. I looked at Will, who was holding up his stickers. "I know those are dolphins," I said. "I couldn't find fish stickers."

4. Will and Viv had a hockey brawl, fighting over who got to put our money into the collection plate. I got hit with an uppercut.

5. When the pastor asked the children what God looked like, Viv's hand shot up. "Half man, half woman," she said. Hermaphrodites R' Us.

6. After partaking in bread and juice for the first time in communion, Will shouted, "What was *that* all about?"

7. On another Sunday, Viv returned to our pew after having communion and announced, "Jesus tastes yummy."

8. The next week, Viv was first up to the communion rail, knelt, and tumbled off in a sideways somersault.

9. While watching a baptism, Will backed up and rear-ended a taller-than-him candle. It was set upright before the entire congregation had to stop, drop, and roll.

10. After saying the Apostles' Creed, Viv turned to me and asked, "What's a virgin, Mom?" Rescue me, Madonna.

One particular Sunday, I started thinking about the ancient ritual of human sacrifice. I was willing to volunteer if it got me out of there faster.

Will, after drawing on both me and the pew, started shooting people with his finger gun. Good to know not allowing him to have toy guns has curbed the allure of firearms.

"Will?" I said. "You can't shoot people in church."

He grinned. I thanked God we didn't name him Dexter.

"Please, Mom?" he said. "Pretty please with butts on top?"

"No shooting people in church. Or I'm taking away every toy you've ever seen."

I fake smiled and tried to listen to what the pastor was saying.

"Mom," Viv whispered. "Look at this."

She had drawn a picture of me. It was pretty good. She had managed to capture my eyes exactly, including every enlarged blood vessel there was.

"It's beautiful," I said.

I started pondering an important religious question: Is sarcasm a virtue or a deadly sin?

I didn't want an answer to that.

HE PUT THE HOSE DOWN THE VENT AND TURNED ON THE WATER

Because I didn't vomit enough during pregnancy, I enjoy stomach-churning rides at amusement parks. As a result, when Viv and Will grew tall enough to go on upside-down rides, I told Chris to take a break. He spent hours with the kids; I'd gladly take them for a solo outing to the fairgrounds.

Viv, my partner in stupidity, took to the Drops of Doom right away. Will was wisely cautious. He'd always been the child who'd survive the Zombie Apocalypse. He'd stay away from the undead and create a manual on how to outsmart them using the 932 facts he knew about carnivores; Viv, meanwhile, would convince the horde of zombies to join her in "Ring Around the Rosie" before she ended up as lunch.

"Come on, Will," I said. "The roller coaster is fun."

"No."

"You can see how it works," I offered.

"No," he paused, "I wish Daddy were here."

"I know you do," I said. "Look, you can sit beside Mommy," I offered. "Viv will sit with a stranger."

"Mom!" Viv said.

"Come on, Will. I'll buy you ice cream if you go on this ride with me."

"A cone?"

"Yes."

"Any flavor?"

"Any."

"OK."

 Parenting Tip: Bribery teaches children important life skills. Like bribery.

And so we lined up for longer than Justin Bieber has been alive, climbed into the roller coaster, and got whiplash while smiling. Despite Will's bug-tooth grin, he never again fell for this bribe.

After Will and Viv enjoyed their cones, we walked to the exit, which meant passing a plethora of games run by underpaid teenagers.

"Can we play this game?" Will asked me, pointing to a game with guns.

"No."

"Why not?" Viv asked.

"Because you don't have a gun license." This is Canada. Parents can harness strict gun laws and use them to control their kids.

"But that girl looks younger than us."

My eyes followed to where she was pointing. "Her parents know the gun license people. She got a special one after she took a course."

"Really?" Will asked.

 Parenting Tip: Twist the laws of your state or country to get your children to obey you.

I pulled them along by their hands, past the basketball hoop shot, the sledgehammer bell game, and the tent filled with Barney-sized stuffed animals.

Finally, we were through the turnstiles. There was no way back.

When we arrived home, I exiled Viv and Will to the backyard so I could start dinner and not ruin the pizza crust. I had told Chris that I would cook something. Following a recipe that reads "add enough flour so the dough isn't sticky but not so much that it is dry" was beyond my remedial cooking abilities. I was pretty sure the technical writers of most recipes worked for IKEA in their early years, writing incomprehensible instructions involving Allen keys, grommets, and other Muppet-sounding terms.

Viv entered the house. "Can Abby and Connor come over?"

"No," I said.

"Why not?"

"Because the last time they were over, Abby got her hair caught in our rope swing, and I had to dial 9-1-1."

"You didn't call 9-1-1; you just called her mom," Viv said.

"She's my 9-1-1," I said.

Abby's dad was a police officer, and her mom was the neighbor who invited me over for wine and informed me about pet stores. That counted as 9-1-1.

"Please?"

"No," I said. "We're having pizza soon."

"You're cooking?" Will asked.

"Yes."

"But Dad always cooks," he said.

"I know he does," I said. "But that doesn't mean I can't do it."

"Can I help?" Viv asked.

"No, thanks."

"Why not?

"Because I'm perfectly capable of wrecking this meal on my own, thank you very much."

"OK." She bounded towards the stairs with her rubber boots still on.

I started rolling the crust, which resembled the state of Texas.

"Mom?" Viv called out.

"Yes?"

"Come look at me."

Her voice came from around the corner, the direction of the stairs. I walked over, peeling the flour-dough mixture from my fingers.

"What are you doing?" I asked. She was in some sort of downward dog position on the stairs. Only she wasn't using her hands.

"I'm climbing the stairs."

"Stop using your head to climb the stairs."

Viv giggled. I smiled.

I walked downstairs to our coffin-sized freezer to get some grated mozzarella. If there was anything that made a homemade tough-crust pizza better, it was adding freezer-burned, pre-grated cheese.

I retrieved it, came upstairs, and heard a rhythmic thudding-squishing sound.

"What are you doing?" I asked Will. He smiled and ignored my question.

Cradling my Ziploc bag of cheese chunks, I watched him. He held the flour-and-dough-covered rolling pin with his right hand and had taken five oranges out of the fruit bowl. He was banging them.

"Are you playing Whac-A-Mole?"

He grinned and continued his orange massacre, his own home version of carnival games.

"Stop. Now. Upstairs. Room." I sighed. "Mommy needs a time out."

He listened. I finished the pizzas, put them in the oven, and cleaned up the carnie-carnage.

Chris came home and gave me a hug.

"You OK?" he said. "Where are the kids?"

"I don't know," I said.

"You don't know?"

"Well, they're upstairs. I just don't know what they're doing."

We heard a thunk. And then some hopping, followed by a thud. We waited in silence for screams that didn't come. Just the voice of Will. "Mom? I'm bleeding." I ran

The first thing I saw was blood dripping from Will's toe onto our beige carpet. Before I could accuse him, he said, "I wasn't even picking my nails, Mom. I cut it on the vent behind the door."

"What we're you doing behind the door?" I asked.

"Trying to listen to you and Dad talk."

Chris joined us upstairs, surveyed the situation, and shrugged. "I'm going to change out of my work clothes," he said. "Need any help?"

"No, thanks. I got it. Really."

I told Viv, who'd already cordoned off the crime scene, to get some tissues. She was out of the blocks faster than Usain Bolt. Then I ordered her to get a Band-Aid.

I returned to Will, sopped up more blood, and found a shallow slice across his baby toe. I got him to sit up so he could bum-scoot to the bathroom, but his toe started bleeding on the carpet again. "Lie down," I said. Given that Will still remembered some of the dog tricks Chris had taught him and Viv years ago, this was an easy command for Will to follow. I wrapped tissues around his toe again, put my hands around his ankles, and dragged him into the bathroom. Despite the rug burn on his back, he found this more enjoyable than the roller coaster.

Viv came back from her Band-Aid quest with one that Chris had purchased at a garage sale. I was pretty sure it was circa 1948. "It's the only one I could find," she said breathlessly. I asked her to get a washcloth. Meanwhile, I let Will bleed onto the linoleum.

Viv returned with a hand towel. "That's not a washcloth," I said. She looked at me quizzically. "A washcloth is smaller." Off she went.

I cleaned and dried Will's cut, applied ointment, and put on the old Band-Aid, which had lost its stickiness. Will, in true Will form, never complained.

I found a newer Band-Aid at the bottom of a gym bag and applied it. I told Will and Viv that we'd had enough excitement for the day. "Just read some books on your beds until the pizza is ready," I said.

I left them, paused to look at the carpet, and went downstairs to tweet this: "How do I get blood out of a beige carpet? #FreakingKids."

Minutes later, I had twelve replies, all saying the same thing: "Peroxide. Now."

I got peroxide from the first aid cupboard and noticed that Viv had destroyed the childproof lock to get to the Band-Aids. I jogged back upstairs. I dabbed. I scrubbed. I finished removing the bloodstain by the time the smoke alarm sounded. The pizza was done.

Parenting Tip: Justify time spent on Twitter as "researching" what is best for your child. Or your carpet.

The next morning, I tried to imbibe enough caffeine to be coherent. Chris, in his caffeine-less state, went downstairs to ensure everything was in order for my parents' visit. They were due to arrive after lunch.

While sipping tea and scanning Twitter, I heard Chris yell. "Lee? Can you come here? It's serious."

I ran down the stairs and found him in the bathroom. The exhaust fan was hanging down, there was water dripping from it, and both Chris and the floor were soaked.

I stared, dumbfounded.

"What the heck is this from?" he asked.

My mind raced, trying to visualize the floor plan of the main level. "Maybe the kitchen sink leaked," I said. "It's right above." I bounded up the stairs, doubling my daily exercise quota, and inspected the sink pipes. No leak.

Then I stopped. *What was on the outside wall?* I wondered.

I ran outside and saw the garden hose lying next to the outdoor exhaust vent that went down to the basement bathroom.

"William!" I screamed as I ran back into the house. He was playing Hot Wheels versus dinosaurs with his peanut-butter-covered fingers.

I assumed my good-cop face, the kind that encouraged kids to confess.

"Yesterday," I paused, catching my breath, "did you put the hose in the vent hole outside?"

"Yes," he said, slamming stegosaurus into a pick-up truck.

"Did you turn the water on?" As if I really needed to ask.

"I think so."

"OK, then. You know that's not a good idea, don't you?" Disciplining is not my strength when I'm on holidays from teaching.

"Sorry, Mom. I won't do it again. I was just doing an experiment," he said. As I went downstairs to sugar coat the news to Chris, I wondered if the mothers of Benjamin Franklin and Albert Einstein had been committed to asylums.

"Well," I told Chris, "the good news is that it's not a leak that needs to be fixed by a plumber."

Chris wrenched his neck out from under the sink. "What is it then?"

"Not *it*," I said, "but *who*."

"Will?"

"Yes," I said. "He put the hose down the vent and turned on the water."

"He *what*?"

"Yup," I said. I knew Chris had heard me. "I talked to him about it. It seems he was conducting his own science experiment."

Chris got up off the floor. "What is this," he said, "National Euphemism Day?"

I laughed. "You have to admit that *science experiment* sounds nicer than *flooded our basement*."

Chris shook his head.

I continued talking. "Look. At least he turned off the hose. It could have been worse. Like the time he left the hose on for two days."

"True enough. And there's no one thousand dollar water bill this time."

"Hey, don't forget the company forgave us that," I said. "Look, I'll clean it up, and I'll get Will to help."

"Don't bother," Chris said. "I have to figure out a way to get all the water out of the vent. I'm pretty sure there's an elbow joint in there."

"Right, OK," I said, pretending I knew what that meant. "I'll just go actually *watch* the kids until Mom and Dad get here."

THE NEXT TIME YOU COME OUT OF THAT ROOM, YOU'D BETTER BE BLEEDING

My dad sat in the time-out chair in our living room. He hadn't done anything wrong, but I suspected it was as far away from chaos as he could get.

Will and Viv wrestled in the middle of us. It was cute for the first round, but each progressive round, they added some new mixed martial art to their attack repertoire. Thai kickboxing was the latest.

Dad watched them with a slight grin. I suspected that he was remembering his days of growing up unsupervised on a farm with four brothers, all competitive. Was he thinking about the time they made homemade grenades from gunpowder they'd found in an abandoned building? Or was he remembering racing cars on the frozen river behind his farmhouse?

My reverie was interrupted by the sound of a foot hitting a rib.

"OK, that's enough," I said.

I had spent six years as a parent cultivating my authority, which was now on par with that of a gnat.

Viv and Will progressed to ground fighting. "Stop it." I took a deep breath and changed tactics. "Let's play a game."

Will released the headlock he had on his sister. "Can we play *What Am I?*"

Viv squealed. "Can I go first? Can Grandma and Grandpa play? Please?"

I looked at my parents. My mom smiled; she'd do anything. My dad, his football build still evident decades later, looked skeptical.

"We'll see," I said, buying us some time. "Viv, you start."

Viv hopped around the room.

"Frog!" Will yelled.

"Nope."

"Bunny," I offered.

"Nope." More maniacal hopping entertained us. Viv paused to put a teddy bear down the front of her pants and proceeded to hop again.

"Kangaroo!" Will shouted.

"Yes," Viv said, as she performed a Caesarean section on herself to rescue the stuffy.

Chris went next. Lying on his back on the couch, he stuck his legs and arms straight out toward the ceiling and feigned sleep.

"Sloth," both kids said, disappointed that Daddy's acting repertoire was limited to this slow-moving beast.

Will took his turn. He strutted around the living room walking like an ancient Egyptian who was nodding his head relentlessly.

"Rooster?" Viv said.

"I was going to say *cock*," Chris said.

My parents laughed. After ten years, they were used to their son-in-law's sense of humor. In fact, I was pretty sure my mom's giggles had turned to silent tears, a frequent occurrence when she enjoyed a double entendre joke.

"I've got one," my dad said.

I paused. I'd never seen my dad play a game that wasn't cribbage.

He stepped into the middle of the carpet, bent his big frame over, pointed an elbow to the ceiling, and did some sort of shuffle. Whatever he was doing, it was convincing.

Will and Viv shouted out the names of random animals, including camels, elephants, and warthogs.

My dad added a few variations. He was in character, and he was doing this animal justice.

Finally, after more guessing, I spoke for the room. "I give up."

Dad sat back down. "It was a killdeer."

There was a pause, before looks of confusion from the kids and laughter from the adults.

"I never knew killdeers had pointy elbows," I said.

"Grandpa?" Will asked. "What's a killdeer?"

"It's a bird," he said, possibly disappointed that his suburban descendants would deign to ask this. "A type of plover," he added.

"Of course it is." I wasn't about to admit I thought a plover was a type of tractor we used in the 1970s.

"I was doing their broken wing act. It's what killdeers do when predators are around."

"And you did it well, Dad." I said. "Want another beer?"

On the second night of my parents' visit, all went well enough. Even Chris was low key, neither burping the alphabet for the kids nor suggesting to Viv that the next book she should get from the library should be *Junie B. Jones Robs a Bank and Flees to Mexico*. By the time bedtime rolled around, Will decided he wanted to kiss only Grandma and me goodnight. *Fair enough*, I thought.

Will cuddled up to me on one side of the couch. Viv glued herself to my mom on the other side. I noted that a restraining order might be in effect if my mom decided she wanted to shower or sleep.

I thought I'd double check on the hug/kiss situation.

"Are you sure you don't want to kiss Grandpa or Daddy goodnight?"

Will looked at my tall father and shook his head. Then he leaned in and whispered something to me.

After wiping saliva from my ear canal, I repeated what I thought I heard. "You want Daddy to kiss Grandpa goodnight for you?"

I started to laugh. So did the other adults.

Will nodded.

"Well," I said to Chris, "are you going to kiss Grandpa?"

"I don't know," he said. "I'm not really a whiskers man."

"And he does give nasty whisker rubs," I added, remembering the playful torture sessions of my childhood.

"How about a handshake, Willy?" my dad asked.

I watched two of the men in my life grasp palms and say goodnight.

I managed to pry Viv away from my mom and followed my kids upstairs to witness them brush their teeth in fewer than ten seconds. I read them Doreen Cronin's *Dooby Dooby Moo* for the 184th time. It was one of the few books I still loved reading aloud, mostly because it let me unleash my inner Steppenwolf.

I tucked them in, kissed them goodnight, and channeled my inner English teacher by quoting Shakespeare: "May flights of angels sing thee to thy rest." I turned out the light and returned to the land of Adultville.

Dad had the cribbage board out, Mom had uncorked a bottle of wine, and Chris came over to squeeze my shoulder before begging off to watch one of his favorite sports teams lose. I knew I had to give him a break since he cheered for the Toronto Maple Leafs, the Toronto Blue Jays, and the Toronto Raptors. The guy hadn't seen a championship in more than a couple of decades. But he's a faithful one, so he watches. I suspected it helped him practice his swearing.

I took a sip of wine and cut the cards. A King. I lost the chance to deal. Mom and Dad talked about the weather and the latest curling bonspiel. I stared at the cribbage board, trying to remember the rules. It was one thing to forget how a killdeer defended itself from its predators; it would be an entirely bigger disappointment if I forgot the rules of cribbage, a game I'd played with my parents since I was in first grade.

My concentration was interrupted. "Mom?" Will said.

"What are you doing up?" I asked. "Go back to bed."

"Mom?" Will repeated. He showed me one of his twenty-two books on dinosaurs.

"Go. To. Bed."

My dad shuffled the deck of cards and dealt.

"Just one question, Mom."

"One," I said.

"What's your favorite dinosaur?"

"You came downstairs to ask me that?"

"Yes."

"It's Leave-Me-Alone-A-Saurus."

My parents laughed. So did Will. "Mom, that's not a real dinosaur. Your favorite is Stegosaurus. You like the plates and the spikes. They help keep Stegosaurus warm when he needs it and cold when he needs it."

"If you knew that, why did you come down to ask?"

Will shrugged. "Goodnight." He ran back upstairs.

I picked up my cards, one of those impossible hands that upped the odds I'd be skunked by my parents.

We started playing. Halfway through that first hand, more little feet. Not to be one-upped by her brother, Viv snuck downstairs and squirmed her way onto my mom's lap.

Mom, Dad, and I finished the first hand. I was losing by ten already.

"OK, Viv," I said. "I know Grandma is loving this—"

I watched them snuggle even closer.

"—but it's bedtime. Up you go."

She trudged upstairs.

We dealt another hand and finished our glasses of wine. I heard the kids' bedroom door squeak open.

I was going to be proactive on this one. "The next time you come out of that room," I yelled, "you'd better be bleeding."

I heard the upstairs door squeak closed. My mom shuffled the cards while my dad filled my wine glass. They understood. They'd been there.

I LOVE THE SOUND OF VACUUMING UP LEGO IN THE MORNING

When I was pregnant, someone gave me a CD called *Mozart for Babies*. I didn't play it. First of all, Mozart wasn't even alive when I got pregnant. Second, Mozart was more popular when he was dead. Third, I preferred Bach. "

Although our musical tastes weren't classical, Chris and I still exposed our kids to a lot of genres. When I wasn't in the vehicle, Chris tended to crank bands like Public Enemy and DJ Champion, his version of soft rock. On the days I played taxi driver to my pair of kids, I'd put the radio on scan and let it cycle around uselessly, mirroring the brain cells in my head, or at least the ones I hadn't killed yet. Every third song, Will would shout, "Stop. This is my second favorite song."

This time, when the snow was falling softly, that song was Lady Gaga's anthem, "Born This Way."

Both Will and Viv knew the words. Every. Single. One.

I concentrated on using my remaining brain cells to focus on driving. It didn't work. If the distracted driving laws were to be fully effective, they'd have to ban driving with children.

Parenting Tip: If you drive with children in the car, you drive distracted. Muzzling and tethering are two options.

In spite of myself, I listened to the lyrics, which were about lipstick and boudoirs.

I focused on not rear-ending the car in front of me.

Then more lyrics sung by my own off-key duo. I heard the words "drag" and "queen" over and over again.

"Where did you learn all the words to Lady Gaga?"

"At school," they chimed. That would be Catholic school. Then again, Gaga attended Convent of the Sacred Heart School, which could likely out-Catholic my kids' school.

I joined Viv and Will for the song's end. When that ended, I waited for the next one. Neil Young. One of his classics: "Heart of Gold." I let the song play. I was a sucker for poetic lyrics; if the singing was atonal, I identified even more. Hello, Leonard Cohen.

I used the steering wheel for a drum and sang along using my own atonal talents: "I've been in my mind, it's such a fine line, That keeps me searching for a heart of gold, And I'm getting old."

Viv said, "I don't like this song. Can you change it?"

Will piped up. "That singer sounds like Shaggy from *Scooby Doo*."

I paused. I may have hit the SUV in front of me. "Pardon me?"

Will repeated, "He sounds like Shaggy. You know? From *Scooby Doo*?"

I lectured my rearview mirror. "Neil Young does not sound like Shaggy from *Scooby Doo*."

"Yes, he does," Vivian said.

Then I smiled as my overworked, remaining cells played a convincing mash up of Neil Young and Shaggy in my brain.

I shut off the radio because it had started to snow more heavily. Some countries might have called it a blizzard; we called it winter.

Snow may be the best free toy ever, but if you're a parent, it's the devil incarnate. Snow looks pretty, much like pregnancy does from a distance. Upon lengthy examination—or personal experience—it loses its appeal and becomes mundane, unpleasant, and vomit inducing.

At the start of every winter, we bundled up Viv and Will in snow pants that were too small, mismatched mittens that doubled as sponges, and scarves that could hang our children on our secondhand swing set. Then, I hoped that my frozen Garden of Eden tableau would last, that I would enjoy ten minutes of silence as my offspring frolicked in our fenced patch of suburban wonderland.

Like that ever happened.

Instead, on a lazy Saturday morning, I drank a cup of tea and listened to muffled yells, trying to classify them into some sort of screaming taxonomy for children, ranging from I-Think-They're-Just-Laughing to Call-a-Coroner.

Somewhere in the middle of that taxonomic rank was a muffled scream, the one that sounded like your child had no tongue. I heard pounding on our patio door followed by words. "Mom? Will's tongue is stuck to the swing post, and he can't move it."

I briefly recalled getting my own tongue stuck to my frosted window as I waited for the yellow school bus to come one morning when I was "little." Age fourteen. It hurt less than my earlier monkey bar incident.

I slipped on my boots and ran outside jacket-less.

"Ahm," Will attempted to enunciate my name. "I -ung ih huck."

"I know your tongue is stuck," I said. "Can you just tear it off?"

He shook his head and then screamed.

"God help me, Will," I muttered, trying to compose myself. "Didn't you learn anything from licking the minivan?"

"Orry."

"OK," I said. "Stay still." I could see my breath. "Vivian?" I yelled. "Bring me a small glass of water. Leave your boots on. Just get it. Now."

"Is Will thirsty?" she asked.

"Just get it."

I leaned my head closer to Will's tongue and started panting like a dog, hoping that my bad breath would melt the ice or at least knock him out. Evidently, the image of his mother bent over blowing on the swing set was too much. Will started to laugh and in the process ripped his tongue off the swing pole.

> Parenting Tip: Making your child laugh is a good way to get his tongue unstuck from a frozen swing set.

"Ow."

I started to laugh.

"It's not funny," he said.

"No, it's not. But Mommy panting like a dog was a bit funny, wasn't it?"

He smiled. I escorted him into the house, where we were met by Viv who was carrying a glass of water.

"Thanks, Viv," I said, taking it. "Drink up, Will."

He drank. "Blood tastes funny," he said.

I removed his boots and grabbed the glass so he could peel off his snow pants. I could see his tongue rolling around his mouth.

Then he spit.

I was just out of range.

Blood spattered everywhere, onto the table, the wall, the floor. It missed the carpet by two inches.

"Stop that!" I yelled. "Don't get blood on the carpet."

It had taken Chris and I months to pick out an area rug that we both didn't hate. The last thing I wanted to do was to peroxide the heck out of it.

I mopped up the blood and the snow that had melted off Viv's boots. Then, because it was the logical thing to do after you mopped the floor, I decided to vacuum. There were enough Cheerios under the table to drive up the price of oats.

When Will and Viv heard the word "vacuum," they picked up their toys quickly. We'd conditioned them, convincing them we'd suck up any homeless toy.

Not long after I started hoovering, it happened. That pleasant sound that secretly pleases every mother. The sound of LEGO being sucked up the hose.

"Mom?" Will screamed, hitting a high taxonomic level. "Was that LEGO?"

I feigned innocence. Then I sucked up another piece.

"Stop, Mom, stop."

I shut off the vacuum cleaner.

"Mom, I missed some LEGO. Stop."

"I love the sound of vacuuming up LEGO in the morning."

"Mom. Stop. Now."

Because the screams of my scabby-tongued son were reaching the Call-the-Coroner levels, I waited and watched him crawl under the chair and rescue a couple of LEGO swords.

"OK," he said, resigned. "Go ahead now."

I'LL SMUGGLE SOME PINOT GRIGIO IN THE KIDS' WATER BOTTLES

Winter passed, bringing us the season of soccer and the challenge of two kids playing on two different teams at two different fields. I had enough equipment to warrant a U-Haul rental. Chris was working, and I struggled as always in my attempt to get everything and everyone out the door. I sent Viv and Will outside while I gathered the last of the gear, which included my mittens and sunglasses. Nothing said soccer season in Canada like contrasting accessories.

I rushed outside and noticed Viv and Will collecting rocks on the side of our driveway.

I loaded the last of the stuff in the back of our minivan and walked around to open Will's door.

I saw this etched on his door: "William." A sad face sat atop his name.

"What the—" I started, not bothering to finish my sentence. "Did you use rocks to write on the—? You couldn't have, could—?"

Viv looked at me. I could tell she was stalling. It was the stealing-pens-from-Staples incident all over again. "I'll crawl in Will's side," she said.

"No. No. You didn't write—" I interrupted myself again. "Did you carve things too?"

I raced to the other side.

I read this: "Vivian only." There were scratches to the left of her name, where she must have tried to get the rock to work properly.

I gasped. Then I saw more. On the rear side-panel of the van, Viv inscribed her etchings. More precisely, she composed a dedication: "on behalf of my class."

My kids knew by my speechlessness that they'd done wrong. I clutched my hair.

I rubbed my index finger across one of the gorges. "This won't come off," I said. "Ever."

I heard choruses of "I'm sorry" and "We didn't know."

And I thought, *Chris is going to freak*. Will and Viv predicted this on their own.

They started crying. "Daddy is going to be so mad, isn't he?"

"Yup."

I drove them to their respective fields, and I popped back and forth to watch them go through the motions in soccer.

When we arrived home, Chris's car was in the garage.

We stood outside and rehearsed how to tell him.

We walked in. They hid behind me in the kitchen.

"Now," I said.

Both kids shook.

"Daddy, we're sorry . . ."

I saw Chris twitch.

"We made a big mistake . . ."

More twitching.

"We used rocks . . ."

Steam.

" . . . and carved our names into the van's paint."

Chris paused, processing this. He sighed, audibly relieved. "I thought you were going to say you wrecked my flat screen TVs," he said.

"You're not annoyed?" I asked. I could barely handle the first shock; this one threatened to send me to a chair. Chris recovered, but never freaked out. *I clearly underestimate this man*, I thought. I grounded the kids for a week. Chris supported my decision. The etchings remain on the van to this day.

It took me a while to get to sleep that night. I tried not to panic as I recalled my insomniac state a year ago. Morning came, and I was in bed drifting in and out of a sluggish weekend slumber. Chris had left for work at some insane hour, leaving me to lie in bed with Viv cuddled into my side and Will snuggled in the nest I'd made with my feet. Because of my industrial-strength earplugs, I couldn't hear the cartoon marathon that played on TV.

Of course, if it started as a perfect morning, there had to be a moment when you free fall from heaven's gates. That moment came just after Will asked for a turn using the remote control. Viv listened. She launched the remote at his head with an accuracy that could make her the answer to the Blue Jays' bullpen problems.

Will didn't cry, but he did complain. He was rubbing his forehead when I pressed my face off my pillow. I removed one of my earplugs. Viv didn't apologize.

So, I did what every parent who's sleep and caffeine deprived does. I overreacted.

"Vivian," I snapped. "Say you're sorry."

She looked at me with wonder.

I took this as defiance. "You can't whack someone in the head and not say you're sorry."

Demonstrating the for-every-action-there-is-reaction principle, she took my anger-induced fastball and knocked it over the fence with a single swing, which—in this case—meant stomping out of the bedroom and slamming the door.

I drifted back to sleep.

Sometime later, I took out my second earplug and yelled again. "Viv? You OK?"

"Yes."

I grabbed five more minutes of sleep before I showered.

When I came out of the bathroom, Viv sat on the edge of my bed, a homemade book in her hand.

I read the title: *Why Don't You Love Me Mom?*

I knew I was in for it.

I read:

Mom doesn't love me.
Oh how can that be?
I wish she would love me.
Just like a new tree.
I just don't know why
I can't make her cry.
But my mom doesn't love me with glee.
My mom isn't the same
With nothing to blame.
I wish she would love me with glee.
Please love me.
Please love me.
Please love me.
Please love me.

Please love me.
Please love me.
Please love me.
Please love me.
Please love me.
Please love me.
Please love me.
Please love me.
Please love me.
Please love me.
Please love me.
Pretty please?
Mom?

After silently reading Viv's book, I did what any mom with half a heart would do: I gave her a hug and defended myself, debate-style.

Before I could get to my second rebuttal, Viv interrupted me.

"Mom," she said, "you have a booger in your nose."

"Right," I said, readjusting my sopping towel so I could grab a Kleenex with an ounce of dignity.

After blowing my nose, I reassured Viv that I loved her forever and for always.

She was not happy to hear this. She looked up at me and said, "You mean I made this book for nothing?"

"Not really," I said, stalling.

"I even Googled 'how to make your mom love you,'" she said.

"You did? What were the results? What should you do to make your mom love you?"

"You should make your mom a craft."

"You did better than that."

"I did?"

"You made me a book. That is 152 times better than a craft that would eventually go to recycling heaven. We definitely need to show this to Daddy."

To make up for my inadequate parenting, we took the kids to the beach. This seemed like a good idea until I developed an allergic reaction to the sun that had me lying on the cold tile on the bathroom floor of my basement the next two nights, trying to soothe the itchy blisters and not sell my soul to the first eBay bidder.

Prior to Operation Allergic Reaction, Will wanted to swim in the lake with me. Now, I'm more of a jump-off-a-dock woman than a wade-into-the-cold-July-Canadian-water woman. Worse, there were sandbars, which meant it took me longer to get wet than it took Octomom to remember her kids' names.

"Can't you just play with Daddy some more?" I asked.

"Mom," Will said. "You have to come into the water at least once."

While Chris built a sandcastle with Viv, my son and I held hands and waded into the lake. Amid the onset of hypothermia, I thought of Virginia Woolf, who had waded into waters with stones in her pockets. Thankfully, I was a long way from that.

Will broke my depressing reverie. "Look, Mom," he said. "The water is up to your pagina."

I laughed. "And the water is way past your venis."

"Mom," he said. "It's penis, not venis."

"You're right. And it's vagina. Not pagina."

"You don't have a pagina then?" he asked.

I shivered again. The water lapped at my belly button, or what was left of my belly button after gestating twins. "No, I don't have a pagina. But I do have a vagina. Repeat after me: V-V-V-Vagina."

We were on our third phonics lesson when I noticed a family floating on an inflatable shark beside us.

"Kind of cold, eh?" I said.

They ignored me like I was Peewee Herman at a matinee.

I dove under. Without stones.

Later that afternoon, a friend asked me to go see a movie. We decided to bring an evening picnic. She suggested dark chocolate and nuts. I suggested wine.

"How will we get it in?" she asked.

"I'll smuggle some Pinot Grigio inside the kids' water bottles."

It was decided. I was bringing the wine, which seemed fitting for *Eat, Pray, Love*. I was excited, not only for the alcohol but for the movie. I had read the book and I actually recognized the names of both lead actors. It was a warm evening, with the sun still high in the sky.

Since I see movies so rarely, I had a paralyzing choice: whether to dress for the outdoor warmth or the indoor air conditioning.

I layered my clothes and opened a bottle of Pinot Grigio, the perfect summer wine, and poured it into my twins' stainless steel sippy cups. I ran upstairs to say goodnight to Viv and Will, grabbed a cardigan, and searched for my keys— my own daily, *Where's Waldo* task. I shouted something to

Chris and then I left, without the two sippy cups filled with alcohol.

My friend and I settled into our seats and broke out our contraband picnic once the previews started. Little napkins, Babybel cheeses, dark chocolate, and wine, wine that was nowhere to be found.

"Crap," I said. "I forgot it on the counter." Then I remembered. "Oh my god, it's in sippy cups." A head movie of my six year olds becoming drunk played in my cortex.

I rushed out of my seat, making everyone in our row stand, tripped on a step, and was dialing home on my cell phone before I hit the lobby.

"Have the kids had anything to drink?" I asked Chris.

"Yeah, they've had a drink," he answered. I could hear his voice tense.

"What did they drink?" I asked

"Are you OK?"

"Did they drink from their sippy cups?"

"I don't know."

"Do they seem drunk?"

"Drunk?"

"I put wine in their sippy cups to bring to the movie."

"You what?"

"I filled them with wine. To smuggle it. But I forgot it on the counter."

"You put wine in their sippy cups?"

"Yes. The stainless steel ones."

I could hear him descending the stairs, cell phone in hand.

"It's still here," he said.

"Can you put it in the fridge?"

"Really?"

"Just put it in a bag first . . . and hide it. I'll have it later."

We hung up. I'm not sure what he agreed to do. I just knew that I'd staved off trying to explain this conundrum to Child and Family Services.

I returned to the movie, feeling light.

I was healthy. I was laughing. I had a husband who not only loved me senselessly, but also liked me. I had healthy children. And I was away from them.

THE SAPPY FILES, PART 6 (OR WHY MY KIDS' THERAPISTS SHOULD HAVE A DRINK, UNLESS THEY'RE ALCOHOLICS, IN WHICH CASE DON'T. BLAME. ME.)

Dearest Will and Viv,

Today you turn seven. Happy Birthday, my darlings.

I hope you think being six has been a lot of fun. You know I'm not good at the big things. I'm not good at planning birthday parties, taking you on a zillion outings (or even two—unless they involve a bookstore and a library), or writing plays for you to act out.

But I think I'm OK at the little things. At laughing at the dinner table, at wrestling, at making music practice manageable by banging my forehead on the keys, at impersonating Donald Duck.

I hope that you will come to see that the little things often matter more than the big ones.

I hope you "get" my writing someday. I'm not going to lie. I write for me. But I also write for you.

I hope that someday you will come to know me as a person in addition to a mom. I hope you will realize that—in spite of my many, many failings—I love you "across my howt [heart] and back again." I hope you know in your core that I am "a comeback-er woman" as you once declared.

I hope that you will come to understand that while I laugh at you, I laugh more at myself. I hope you'll see this as a gift.

I hope that you know how thankful your daddy and I are for you both.

I hope.

For you.

For me.

For all of us.

And I know.

I know the world is much, much better with you a part of it.

Much love always,

Mom

THE POST-AMBLE
or The Sappy-File
Finale

THE FINAL SAPPY FILE (OR WHY I NEED TO LAUGH)

Dear Younger Me, the barely pregnant one who doesn't yet waddle and whose stomach is stretch mark free:

File this letter in the if-I-only-knew-then category, or in the box of photos you swore you'd put in an album even though no one prints photos anymore.

It's OK to be scared. Anything worthwhile involves risk, and parenting is certainly worthwhile. In fact, if you're not scared, you're likely in denial or drunk.

Once your babies are born, toss out the serious parenting books. OK, save one for reference so when your daughter starts shooting out blue poo, you know it's nor-maall. But don't read how-to-be-better parenting books. If you sincerely wish to be better, talk to parents you admire. Ask them what worked. What didn't. But the books?

Have a bonfire and roast marshmallows over them.

Trust yourself. As my friend Vanessa once told me, "You are your child's best mother." Trust that becoming a mom doesn't mean you'll lose your personality. It's too strong. You're too strong.

Trust others. It's a lot easier to parent with your own village. Let the Coca-Cola delivery man hold your baby. The drunken women too. Maybe. Cautiously.

Laugh. At your babies. At your husband. And especially at yourself. It's a lot easier to forgive when you laugh. In fact, forgiveness—especially of yourself—may not even be possible without laughing at it all.

Know that it's all a stage: the small stuff (like sleeplessness and toxic diapers) and the big stuff (your child's dependence and even your life).

But laugh. Yes, laugh. When you tell your son, "Get that train off your penis" and your daughter, "Don't lick the minivan," laugh. With wild abandon. Make that your new nor-maall.

Love,

Your stretch marked, know-it-all self

ACKNOWLEDGMENTS
or People I Didn't Forget
To Thank

I'd like to hold a moment of silence for all of the letter U's that sacrificed their lives when this book was translated from Canadian to American. U will not be forgotten.

To Jill Marr, my rock star agent, who once said the best part of her job is that she gets to make dreams come true: Thank you for being my fairy godmother and for becoming my good friend.

To Julie Matysik, my editor at Skyhorse: You believed in my manuscript and humour-humor from the beginning. Your positivity is infectious.

I would be nowhere without my Easy Writers Critique Group. To Nancy Hayes, my gentle guide and inspiration: I want to be you when I grow up. To Brad Somer: I apologize for the twenty-eight exclamation points that I left in. There were originally eighty-two. I hope you're proud! To Elena Aitken and Trish Loye Elliott, my wordb*tches, my beta readers, my besties: If it weren't for you two, I wouldn't have believed. Please tell your husbands that "bad mom" thanks them as well.

Every book needs an early reader who has a PhD in Medieval Gynecology. I'm glad Lorraine Valestuk was mine. To Jenny Hansen: I'm sorry reading my manuscript gave you a migraine; you endured. My go-to funny guy is Chase

McFadden, who is talented enough to write for *SNL*. Clay Morgan is my indefatigable writing partner in all things nonfiction. Thank you, my friend.

If ever there was a writer made by a writing conference, it was me. Surrey International Writers' Conference is fabulous.

When I started IronicMom.com, I never knew I'd develop so many friendships. My readers regularly out-funny me and still they come back. I salute them. And to my real-life friends who put up with me and my writing, I owe you.

I'd be remiss if I didn't mention my teaching colleagues and students. I get to work with quirky, imaginative teens and adults every day. I know how lucky I am.

Finally, my family. To Mom, Dad, Patti, and Steve: Apparently not everyone grows up in a family where unconditional love and battles of wit are the norm. To my in-laws: Apparently not everyone marries into a family with a sense of humor and open arms. To my husband Chris: Thank you for believing in the third funniest woman you've ever met and for loving her senselessly. Back at ya, eh? Base camp rocks. And to my VW: For bearing with a distracted mom and for making her better, in every way. I love you all across my heart and back.

And thank you to _____ (insert your name here). You know who you are. At least I hope you do.

RESOURCES
or High Tech-y Stuff

To find reading guides, supplementary material, and general hilarity, visit the following sites:

- IronicMom.com
- Facebook.com/Leanne.Shirtliffe

If you wish to feel all Star Trek-y, just scan this code, which will take you to Leanne's website:

This QR code is a modern-day Rorschach test. If you can see a face in it, call a therapist.

INDEX

or A Completely Unhelpful but Accurate Classification

---

[1] Yes, I overdid the "ceiling fan" references. Consider it a motif, whatever that is.

[2] Not enough references to him, according to my husband.

[3] Too many references to him, according to my husband.